W9-BHU-716

the

YOGI
ASSIGNMENT

ALSO BY KINO MacGREGOR

The Power of Ashtanga Yoga I

The Power of Ashtanga Yoga II

the
YOGI
ASSIGNMENT

A 30-DAY PROGRAM *for* BRINGING
YOGA PRACTICE *and* WISDOM
to YOUR EVERYDAY LIFE

KINO MacGREGOR

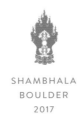

SHAMBHALA
BOULDER
2017

Shambhala Publications, Inc.
4720 Walnut Street
Boulder, Colorado 80301
www.shambhala.com

© 2017 by Kino MacGregor
All rights reserved. No part of this book may be reproduced in any form
or by any means, electronic or mechanical, including photocopying,
recording, or by any information storage and retrieval system,
without permission in writing from the publisher.
9 8 7 6 5 4 3 2 1

First Edition
Printed in the United States of America

♾ This edition is printed on acid-free paper that meets the
American National Standards Institute Z39.48 Standard.
♻ Shambhala Publications makes every effort to print on recycled paper.
For more information please visit www.shambhala.com.

Distributed in the United States by Penguin Random House LLC
and in Canada by Random House of Canada Ltd

Designed by Allison Meierding

Library of Congress Cataloging-in-Publication Data

Names: MacGregor, Kino, author.
Title: The yogi assignment: a 30-day program for bringing yoga practice and wisdom to
your everyday life / Kino MacGregor.
Description: Boulder, Colorado: Shambhala Publications, Inc., 2017.
Identifiers: LCCN 2016045164 | ISBN 9781611803860 (pbk.: alk. paper)
Subjects: LCSH: Yoga. | Meditation. | Mind and body.
Classification: LCC RA781.67 .M33 2017 | DDC 613.7/046—dc23 LC record available at
https://lccn.loc.gov/2016045164

I DEDICATE THIS BOOK TO EVERY SINCERE STUDENT OF YOGA.
I believe in yoga, but more important, I believe in *you*. You
are a generation of yogis, and you are changing the world.
Without you, this book would not be possible.

I give special thanks to my best friend and Instagram yoga
challenge partner-in-crime, Kerri Verna, whom many of you
know as Beach Yoga Girl. Kerri, you are the most authentic
yogi I have ever known.

Thank you to the most talented photographer and filmmaker,
Agathe Padovani, who can make any situation anywhere
in the world look beautiful. All photos in this book are the
result of Agathe's genius eye for beauty.

An infinite debt of gratitude to my teachers, Shri R. Sharath Jois
and Shri K. Pattabhi Jois, without whom I would never have
had the strength to practice. And special thanks to Ajay Tokas
for being an emergency Sanskrit reference.

I am ever grateful to my husband, Tim Feldmann, for
the miracle of his undaunted love of this overachieving,
hand-standing, little fireball. I would be lost without my
mom, whose boundless energy, enlightened perspective,
and sense of humor always shine through on a rainy day.
And I honor my dad, the kindhearted man who raised
orchids and Dobermans and has done nothing but love me
my entire life—I miss you already, Dad, and I love you more
than the universe.

Contents

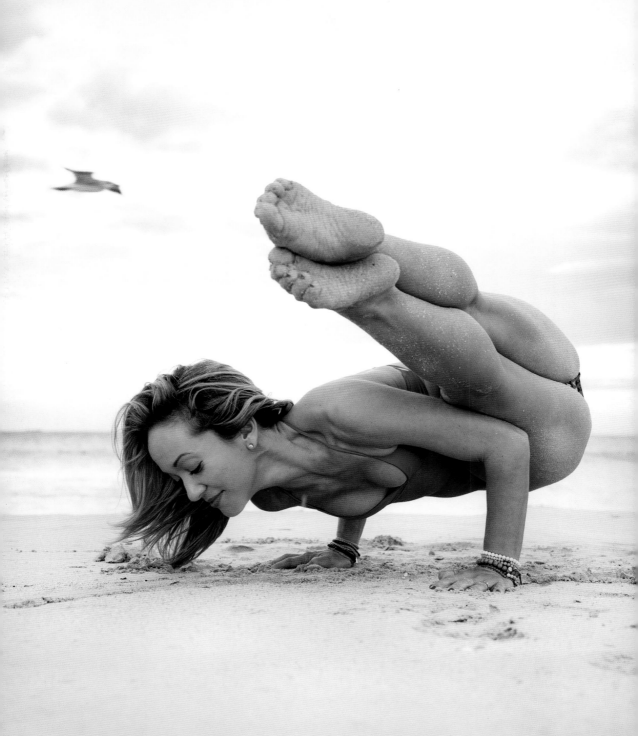

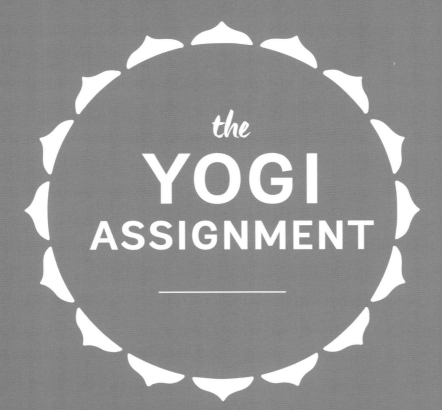

the
YOGI
ASSIGNMENT

_____

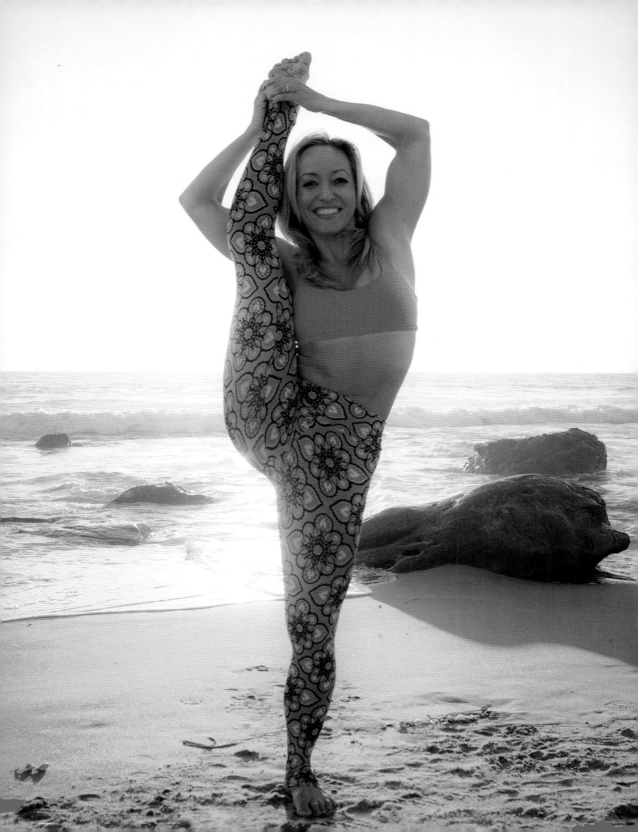

Introduction
Welcome to the Yogi Assignment

I am about to ask you to take a yoga journey with me that may be the most challenging—but also the most unique and fulfilling—practice adventure that you have yet experienced in your yoga life. It's going to require you to be patient when you're not, to let go of negativity when you're simmering with anger, to quiet the voice of judgment in your head toward yourself or someone else, and to exhibit kindness and generosity when you feel unable to do that. Between traffic jams, travel delays, dirty dishes, barking dogs, screaming babies, bills to pay, laundry piles, and the thousand other things that are on your to-do list, it will not be easy to focus and systematically embody the values and precepts of yoga as much as possible in your daily life. But that is what I'm asking you to do.

Most people associate yoga practice with asanas, or postures and sequences, and that is a key part of the tradition. But it is just one part. The benchmark of yogic values and precepts is set in Patanjali's Yoga Sutras. Writing more than two thousand years ago, the sage Patanjali outlines the path of yoga in its totality over a series of four books and 196 aphorisms. There is a wealth of information about the inner journey of yoga, but not one sutra discusses asana technique. Instead, Patanjali presents yoga as a spiritual path of awakening that leads to the goal of a steady, calm, and equanimous mind. The name *Ashtanga Yoga* comes from the second book of the Yoga Sutras, in which Patanjali outlines the eight-limbed path of yoga. *Ashtanga* is formed from the Sanskrit words *astau* ("eight") and *anga* ("limbs"). The eight limbs of Ashtanga Yoga are as follows:

1. Moral and ethical guidelines that define the yogi's relationship with society (*yamas*)
2. Moral and ethical guidelines that define the yogi's personal observances (*niyamas*)
3. Physical poses (*asanas*)
4. Breathing (*pranayama*)
5. Sense withdrawal (*pratyahara*)
6. Concentration (*dharana*)

7. Meditation (*dhyana*)

8. Ultimate peace (*samadhi*)

Beyond that, the yamas and niyamas each contain five subcategories to form a holistic foundation for the yogi's life. The yamas are defined as

1. Nonviolence (*ahimsa*)

2. Truthfulness (*satya*)

3. Nonstealing (*asteya*)

4. Sexual Restraint (*brahmacharya*)

5. Nonpossessiveness (*aparigraha*)

The niyamas are as follows:

1. Purity (*saucha*)

2. Contentment (*santosha*)

3. Discipline (*tapas*)

4. Study (*svadhyaya*)

5. Surrender to God (Isvara *pranidhana*)

So, within the traditional presentation of the values and precepts of yoga, asana is merely one limb of the eight-limbed path.

After nearly twenty years of Ashtanga Yoga practice, I now measure my success by how long I'm able to keep my emotional center spacious enough to be genuinely kind. By comparison, it's almost easy to get on the mat and bend and twist your body. In daily life, it is much harder to maintain a kind and generous heart in the face of adversity and stress. The purpose of every yoga pose is really to present you with a microcosm of your life—both the positive and the negative experiences. We need just as much training in how to be at peace with difficulty as we do in how not to get too attached to happiness. The brave heart of a yogi is defined by actions that make the world a better place. All the effort you pour into asana is really just a testing ground for the effort you will have to exert to apply the yogic values and principles in real life. Yoga is a physical discipline with a spiritual intention. The power of the postures lies not in their masterful execution but in the journey on which each asana takes you.

Each pose has a lesson to teach, and that lesson has very little to do with the flexibility of your hips or the power of your lift. Instead, the spiritual lesson of each asana is always about being kind and generous in spirit.

This book is a thirty-day personal and spiritual challenge. I have distilled some essential teachings of yoga to thirty key lessons that will help you live the yogi's life. Each day will begin with a discussion of the Yogi Assignment and include a few life applications and yoga poses for personal practice. You will find a selection of poses in the pose glossary on page 218, which you can refer to as needed. Each day is actually a journey in itself and should push you to question your emotional, physical, and mental limitations. It is my hope that these thirty days of Yogi Assignments will elicit hope and change in your life.

The inspiration to write this book came from my social media. After hosting monthly yoga challenges on Instagram for a few years, I was encouraged to give out daily Yogi Assignments across all my social platforms. Each morning I searched for a poignant and essential lesson on the yoga path and then shared it across Instagram, Snapchat, and Periscope and sometimes on YouTube. It was then that I realized that living the yogi's life is the real yoga challenge.

Taking on the task of being kind all day, speaking only truthful statements, or remaining calm and equanimous in the face of difficulty may feel like an insurmountable goal and one that, much like the Ashtanga Yoga method itself, we will never accomplish in its entirety. While I am by no means a Vedic or Sanskrit scholar, I find myself at a unique place in the yoga tradition. With one foot in the ancient Indian practice and the other foot in the Western material world, this book is very much a reflection of me. My life and teaching are an example of what it means to live the yogi's life as a contemporary person engaging in the digital age. I hope you will take on the mantle of yoga as a spiritual path, carry it forward to future generations, and make the whole world a more peaceful place.

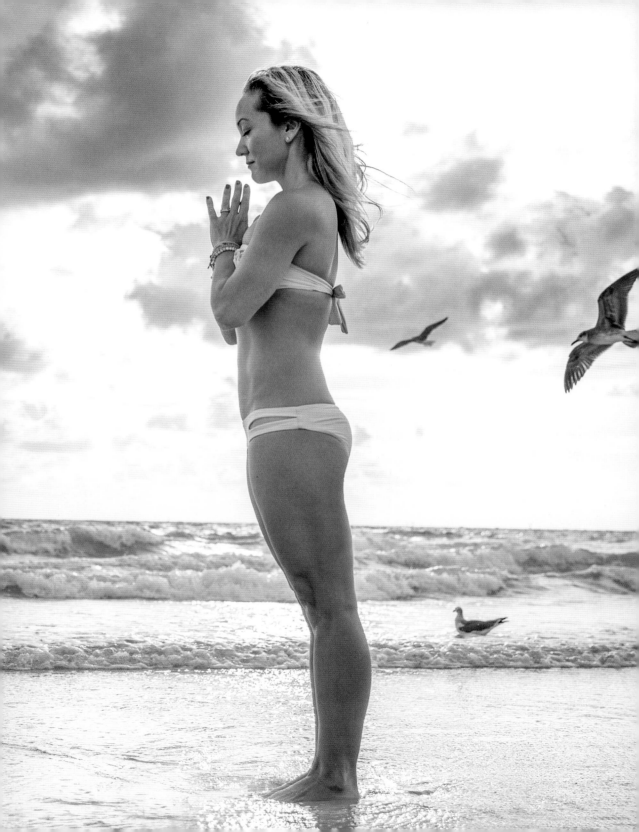

Stillness
Nirodah

When I first started practicing yoga, I attempted to prove my worth through the accumulation of poses. I took the materialistic mind-set that had defined my life into my yoga practice. Instead of getting a sense of self-worth from the accumulation of wealth or assets, I measured myself by how many poses I could do. But since my sense of self-worth was tied to the poses, I falsely assumed that the more advanced the poses I mastered were, the more enlightened I would be. I was never calm when I practiced because I felt like my whole life depended on the poses. If I succeeded in Headstand, then I felt like a good person and had a good day, but if I failed at Headstand, then I felt like a bad person and had a bad day. This set me off on an emotional roller coaster. And this is simply not yoga.

Believing that the poses will give you some sense of self-worth or that doing an advanced pose proves your spiritual worthiness is a false assumption—and it is a trap into which many yoga practitioners fall. It's a kind of materialism that leads to a state of anxiety and discomfort. Yoga is a spiritual path that is about valuing yourself regardless of the state of your material existence. Basically, you have to learn how to be a good person and have a good day regardless of what yoga pose you happen to succeed or fail at during your daily practice. To break free from the material pursuit of yoga poses, you have to become still and discover the true self within.

The choice between the spiritual and the material is an epic battle that unfolds in the heart of the yogi every day. It has been chronicled in one of the most ancient stories of yogic heroism known as the Bhagavad Gita. In this part of the Mahabharata epic, the warrior prince Arjuna stands on the field before a crucial battle between the Kurus and Pandavas, which is a metaphor for the battle between good and evil, or the spiritual and the material. He is granted prescience of the day's events through the grace of the divine incarnation of his guide and charioteer, Krishna.

Arjuna sees that he will win at the cost of much death and misery and responds with horror and disillusionment. Arjuna tells Krishna that his victory will be tainted with blood, his mind confused, his heart grief-stricken, and that, quite simply, he will not fight. Then Arjuna becomes still. It is this stillness that allows Krishna to begin the teaching of the path of yoga, on which the remainder of the Gita expounds.

Stillness, quietness of the mind, silence of the voice, is the path to inner listening and inner awareness. It is the essential quality of the yogic aspirant. The story I just recounted, often called "the despair of Arjuna," highlights a pivotal moment of suffering that every yogi faces. When confronted with the overwhelming pain and suffering of life, we want to quit, just as Arjuna did. Yet if we follow his path and become still, we create the space to listen for inner wisdom.

Yoga can be defined as a descent into the true self contained within. Redirecting the organs of the five senses from the external world to the inner realms is the first step toward experiencing stillness of the mind. One way to understand the nature of mind is to think of it as an ocean of consciousness spanning far and wide. What is evident on the surface is only the beginning; the true power of the ocean is revealed in its depths. Only when the waters reach a still point is it possible to gaze farther down. Then, after a sustained period of stillness, it is perhaps possible to see all the way to the ocean floor. Stillness of the mind is the access point to the direct perception of the true self within. Yoga as a philosophy believes that the truth is available to all who seek it. The truth is not some esoteric principle to be kept under lock and key for a select few. Instead, yoga liberates the knowledge of the inner truth and the freedom of a still mind. Now you're joining the legions of yogis who have embarked on the heroic quest for stillness each time you partake in the practice.

In his Yoga Sutra, Patanjali states that yoga is a stilling of the mind. The normal activity of living stimulates the mind and draws our attention outward to the external world. Each time we interact with the world, waves called *vrittis* reverberate on the ocean surface of the mind. A vritti is like a ripple that disrupts the calmness of the mind and can become part of our habitual, unconscious behavior if we are not aware enough to stop it. More vrittis mean more emotions and thoughts, likes and dislikes, that occlude the mind's natural state of clarity. The more we get caught in the cycle of action and reaction based on the external world, the more waves and emotional storms there will be on the sea of our consciousness.

The alternative is the state of *nirodah*, or stillness. By redirecting the mind to the inner experience, you are able to still the waters of the mind and perceive the depth of the inner self. The trained mind, adept in the state of nirodah, recognizes the true nature of the self within and is steady in the face of any difficulties that may arise while traveling the ocean of life. You suddenly realize that you are not your body, your thoughts, your job, or your home. You have a calm inner sanctuary that is the root of your true sense of self. You see yourself through the eyes of spirit. Stillness is your access point to this inner world.

Similarly, there is an inner body just beneath the skin. While it may be easy to think of the body as mere bones, tissues, and fluids, it is actually a reservoir of depth and power. In yoga, it is possible to feel the darkest and most intimate reaches of the body that cannot be seen with the naked eye. What does that feel like? When I first started practice, I felt my body in a gross and unrefined manner. I knew, for example, that I had hamstrings and that they needed to stretch to enter a forward bend. But later, after many years of practice, my entry into a forward bend is defined by the presence of stillness. Instead of stretching my hamstrings, I become still, enter the inner body, and then explore what wants to happen in that quiet space. Sometimes there is an experience of ease and flow around my hip joints so my skeletal structure seems to float in suspension. Sometimes there is a sensation through my legs like waterfalls cascading into the earth under my feet. Sometimes there is a feeling of emptiness and lightness deep in the center of my pelvis. Sometimes there is simply stillness, beingness, and deep peace. If you cultivate stillness as a mental state, you will also find the magical realm of the inner body.

Yoga is a tool that teaches you how to dig down deep enough to get a glimpse of the eternal. In the eternal space of the inner body, some experiences are so deep that they leave you changed forever. This type of moment is a pivotal turning point in your life. You know that moment because you feel in your gut that your life will change. You are stronger, more aware, more yourself, less selfish, but also less interested in pleasing others. The stillness within you is unchanging and eternal, timeless and real, compassionate and fierce.

Yoga gives you the strength to be brave enough to face your deeply held emotions and feel your way through to the deep resolution and acceptance that is stillness. Look and listen with an open heart and a soft, receptive spirit. Trust the stillness within you.

1. Cultivate stillness. Get into a comfortable seated position and close your eyes. Bring your mind's point of attention to your heart center. Feel your sternum and chest from a physical standpoint. Perhaps you feel your clothes making contact with that area. Be aware of your breath as it moves in and out of your lungs. Start off with the real, tactile sensations of your body. As the mind stills, drop your attention into the space beneath the skin and bones of your sternum. Discover the spiritual heart center in the inner body by looking deeply within. As your power of perception deepens, you may become aware of subtler sensations, like heaviness or lightness, or of emotions such as sadness, happiness, anger, or anxiety. Or you may become aware of the presence of infinite depth, pure light, or peace.

Rest your mind here for at least one minute and listen with inner hearing, see with inner sight, feel through the inner body. It doesn't have to be ceremonious or grand. You could simply close your eyes at your computer for one minute or choose to remain in your car for a minute before going in to work or driving home. Or you might choose to sit in a meditation posture. Quiet the mind and listen with no expectation and no attachment. Do this once a day for thirty days and write down your experiences in a journal.

2. Respond with stillness. The next time you feel yourself itching to respond to an annoying situation in your life, pause, close your eyes, and take a few deep breaths without changing your posture before responding.

3. Schedule stillness. If you have a hard time finding the time to be still because of a busy life, schedule five minutes a day of silent reflection. It could be as simple as turning off the music while driving, turning off the TV, closing your laptop, going for a walk around the block, or stopping to look up at the sky periodically. Take five minutes a day of quiet inner reflection. Schedule it in, and honor your appointment.

1. *Samasthiti*—Equal Standing Pose

Stand at the front of your mat with the bases of your big toes together and leave a small space between your heels. Gently engage your quadriceps, activate your pelvic floor, draw your lower belly in, free your shoulders, and allow energy to flow along the central axis of your body. Use prayer position for the hands when holding Samasthiti for chanting or meditation. But relaxing the arms by the side may help release tension. Samasthiti represents the still point from which all movement begins. It is the space between breaths in the present moment, perfectly positioned between future and past. In the space of now, there is a stillness that speaks.

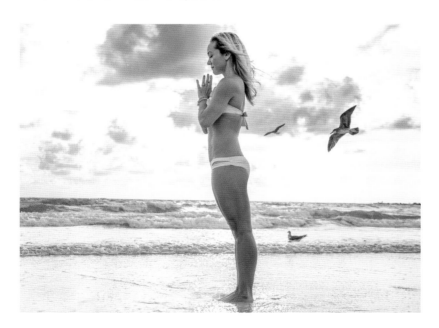

2. *Urdhva Kukkutasana*—Flying Rooster Pose

When you first see this pose, you may wonder how to get into it. The transition requires you to find an inner stillness, although the move-ment itself is not as challenging as it may seem at first. You will need a calm, steady mind to approach this pose. I chose to include Urdhva Kukkutasana because attempting this pose was an emotional journey that taught me strength and stillness of mind. For many years, I felt unworthy because this pose was inaccessible to me. You too may

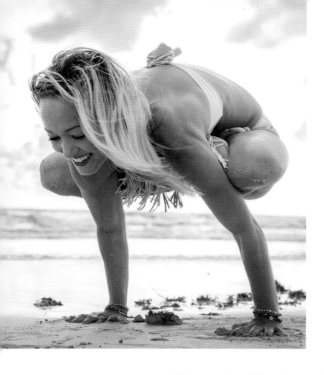

find it very difficult or nearly impossible. Yet if you integrate the impossible into your practice while maintaining a calm, quiet mind, you will become stronger for trying! Never judge yourself by whether you achieve the aesthetic shape of the pose. Go on the inner journey, and let the state of your stillness be your measure of success.

There are many different ways to enter this challenging arm balance. Let's start with the most basic. From a seated position, fold your legs into Padmasana (Lotus Pose). Roll forward onto your knees, and place your hands on the mat directly in front of your knees. Stabilize your shoulders and draw your lower ribs in toward your spine. Tilt your shoulders forward and bend your elbows slightly. Lean to the right to lift your left knee toward your left armpit. Lean toward the left to lift your right knee toward your right armpit. The knees may not actually reach the armpits. As long as the knees rest on the upper arms above the elbow, the pose should be accessible. Straighten both arms and press down firmly from your shoulders. Tighten your core, send your hips back and up, and gaze toward your nose. Stay here for five breaths. Exhale and jump back to Chaturanga Dandasana (Four-Pointed Staff Pose), releasing Padmasana along the way. Note that Bakasana (Crane Pose) can be used as a modification if you cannot do Padmasana yet.

3. *Urdhva Mukha Paschimattanasana*—Upward-Facing Intense Stretch

Urdhva Mukha Paschimattanasana is the upward-facing version of the forward bend known as Paschimattanasana (Deep Forward Fold). This floating forward bend embodies the stillness required to discover the inner body. If you enter it with force and no awareness of the inner space of your pelvis, then the pose is essentially impossible. To practice this pose, you will need a calm, steady mind.

Start in a supine position. Inhale and lift your legs over the top of your head. Touch your toes to the ground behind your head as in Halasana (Plow Pose). Flex your feet slightly and hold on to them near your heels. Exhale to stabilize your pelvic floor. Inhale as you gently roll up to a seated position by rolling up each vertebra. Use your hips to initiate and direct your movement. Keep your legs straight and maintain the same grip on your feet throughout the transition. Find your balance with straight arms and straight legs. Exhale and fold your chest toward your thighs by drawing the head of each down into its socket. If you can't manage the roll-up transition with straight legs, then allow your knees to bend as you come up and straighten your legs as much as possible once you are seated. Stay here for five breaths. Inhale and straighten your arms, exhale and settle into the V-shape pose, and then release your feet, returning to seated.

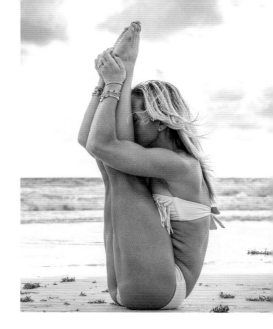

4. *Krounchasana*—Heron Pose

Krounchasana demands a high level of internal rotation. Most internally directed poses help the mind drop deeper into inner awareness and create a reflection on the true self within.

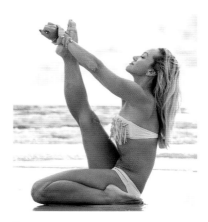

Start in a seated position and fold your left knee back with a deep internal rotation of your left hip; your left foot should be beside your left hip. Drop the head of your right thighbone into its socket as you raise your right leg. If possible, keep your right leg straight as you lift it and clasp your hands around your instep. If your hamstring feels tight, bend your right knee. Inhale to create space and length through your inner body. Exhale as you fold your right leg in toward the center line of your body by continuing to pull downward on your right thighbone. Slowly bring your chin toward the shin or the head to the knee. Align your right knee with your sternum to facilitate a gentle internal rotation and find stillness in the full expression of Krounchasana. Stay here for five breaths. Inhale, straighten your arms, and straighten your head away from your right leg. Exhale to stabilize your pelvic floor, then place your hands on the floor and exit the pose. Repeat on the left side.

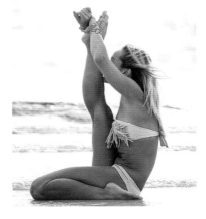

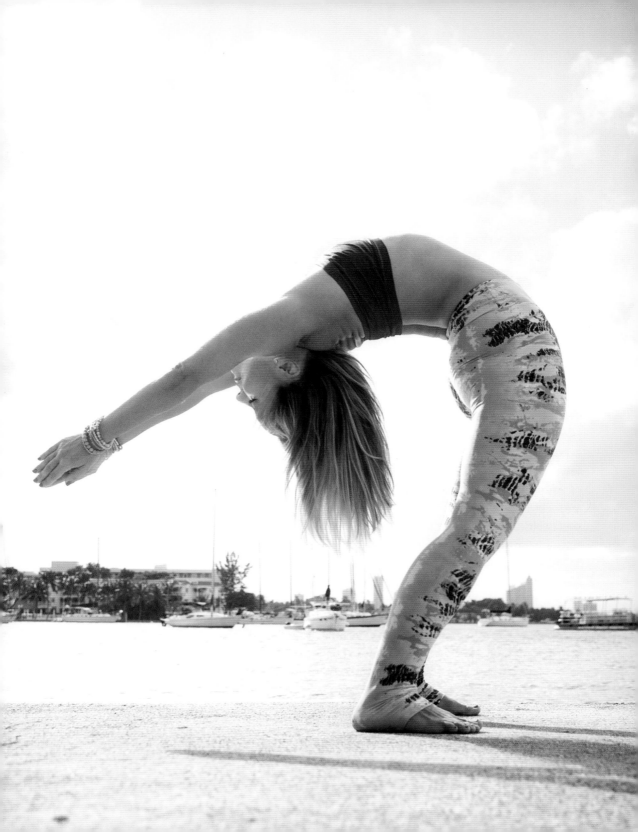

Vulnerability
Arakshitah

Every one of us has experienced trauma to varying degrees, whether physical, relational (or interpersonal), environmental, financial, or some other form. Most often, traumatic experiences leave a kind of emotional scar tissue around the heart, mind, or body. We develop this as protection against the overwhelming feelings of pure panic, sadness, or uncontrollable rage. We stuff our feelings deep inside, turn a blind eye to our vulnerabilities, and build up an emotional armor. These are just temporary measures, however. Feelings of anger and hurt never really go away when we just ignore them. Every emotion you swallow takes up residence in your body and gets stored in the subconscious mind. Those unprocessed emotions are still with you, and they will sometimes bubble up to the surface and disturb the apparently smooth veneer of personality that often protects your inner world.

Many people come to yoga to escape the suffering in their lives and find a more peaceful existence. However, the yoga path is not an escape. Instead, the peace that comes from yoga happens when you truly accept yourself in totality. Yoga "works" when your heart grows so big it can contain the good and the bad, the happy and the sad.

Today's Yogi Assignment is vulnerability, or *arakshitah*. *Arakshitah* means "unprotected" and is best illustrated by the Sanskrit poet Kalidasa's story of the warrior king Dusyanta in the *Recognition of Shakuntala*. A hermit from the Rishi Kanva ashram stops Dusyanta when he is about to kill a deer while on a hunt. The hermit explains that the deer is inviolable because it belongs to the spiritual sanctuary and that the king's weapon must be used to protect the distressed rather than kill the innocent. The king and the deer are juxtaposed as a dichotomy between power and vulnerability, and the hermit yogi counsels that the purpose of power is to honor vulnerability and never harm it. By obeying the hermit, the king passes the test of the deer and is deemed worthy.

Dusyanta then confronts the ultimate vulnerability upon entering the ashram—that is, falling in love. He meets Shakuntala and gives her a royal ring as a sign of their love. This is when Dusyanta becomes spiritually brave.

In the context of yoga, we are both the mighty warrior king and the innocent deer, and our greatest responsibility is navigating our complex roles in life. We have often suffered at the imbalance of power and vulnerability in our lives. Facing our feelings with an equanimous mind and a receptive heart is a crucial step in the healing journey of yoga.

Many yoga poses are specifically designed to make you feel all those emotions that lie dormant, stuffed somewhere in your body. In a sense, many of the asanas act as triggers that stimulate the scary emotions hidden under the surface layer of the superficial self. In the safe space of the yoga practice, you can feel your vulnerability and make peace with yourself. By cultivating a response based on your breathing, posture, and focal point, you learn that you are bigger and stronger than any of your emotions or past experiences.

I've suffered from periods of depression since I was nine years old, and I still sometimes get crippling panic attacks that sabotage my day. Sometimes I cry when I practice, especially after deep backbends. I get flashbacks of things from my past that I thought I had under lock and key in the safety deposit box of my subconscious mind. There are aspects of my childhood that I have tried to forget, things that I never dared to share with others. It took me more than twenty years to be completely honest with myself and another ten years before I even let myself get angry or sad about everything that happened. My response to a series of early childhood sexual traumas was to tell no one and pretend that everything was normal. But I never really had it under control because all that unprocessed sadness and anger came out as panic, narcissism, depression, and drug use. I was afraid to share my secrets because I was afraid I would be rejected and judged. But it was really my own irresolution that prevented me from having the strength to be exactly who I am, complete with my imperfections, and still love myself. Through my practice, I've learned how to let the warrior and the deer become friends.

Tears are no surprise in yoga class. Almost everyone who approaches deeper backbends will at some moment find themselves feeling a weepy sensation welling up from within. As my teacher R. Sharath Jois says, when there are tears, "yoga is working." It is not our perfections that connect us but our vulnerability. It is the tenderness of our broken, cracked hearts that makes us who we are. You are whole and complete, and everything you have experienced is part of a divine plan. You are exactly where you need to be, going through exactly what you need to be going through. Today's practice is to recognize, open up to, and accept your vulnerability—even if it brings you to tears. Share the raw, unedited, unprocessed version of yourself.

HOMEWORK

1. Be vulnerable with yourself. Write in your journal about some difficult moments in your life. Give yourself permission to feel every emotion. Hold nothing back, and be brutally honest. Reconnect to the innocence of the deer within.

2. Be vulnerable with another person. Share one of your secrets with another person, or make a social media post that expresses some aspect of your vulnerability. Share this information without any attachment to or expectation about the response. You are sharing your truth to set yourself free, not to get the approval or acceptance of another person or an online community.

3. Give someone the space to be vulnerable. Ask questions and listen with an open, nonjudgmental heart. Empathize and draw the person out of his or her emotional protection. Channel your inner warrior king and protect the vulnerable space of intimacy.

PRACTICE

1. *Garbha Pindasana/Kukkutasana*—Womb Embryo Pose/
Rooster Pose

These two poses together form one of the most awkward parts of the
practice. Nothing brings out your vulnerability more than flailing around
with your hands stuck between your legs. To attempt Garbha Pindasana
means to risk flopping around like a baby. The dramatic shift from
the vulnerability of this pose to the strength of Kukkutasana is a key
lesson in the yoga path. Taken together, these two poses illustrate the
necessary balance between power and vulnerability.

Start from a seated position and fold your legs into Padmasana.
Draw your legs into your chest and balance on the space between your
sitting bones and your tailbone. Weave your arms through your legs,
start with your right hand. Cup your fingers and aim them toward the
center of your body by gliding them through the space between your
right calf muscle and thigh. Once your elbow clears through your leg,
bend the elbow and draw your right hand up toward your face. Repeat
with your left hand and arm. Use a little water on your skin to lessen the
friction, and consider wearing shorts to make this process easier. Place
both hands under your chin and gaze at your nose for five breaths to
enter Garbha Pindasana. If you cannot slide your hands through your
legs, then simply pull your thighs in toward your chest. If you cannot do
Padmasana, sit with your feet crossed and hold on to the opposite ankle
to pull your legs up.

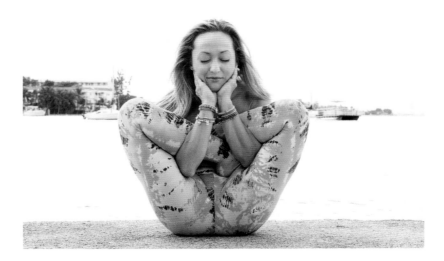

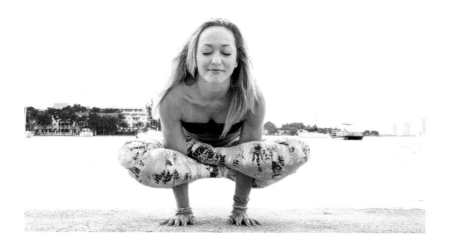

Next, tuck your head down toward your chest and roll back and forth to turn around in a circle on your mat. Exhale as you roll back, and inhale as you roll up. Don't be surprised if you get stuck on your back and end up feeling vulnerable and in need of help. Roll your body from your center of gravity and learn to pick yourself back up. After rocking back and forth five times, reorient toward the front of your yoga mat. Inhale, let go of your chin, and roll forward onto your hands. Allow your thighs to slide down just under your elbows. Inhale as you press down into your hands, stabilize your shoulder girdle, draw your pelvic floor inward, and firm your lower abdominal muscles to lift up into Kukkutasana. If you are modifying the pose, simply place your hands on the ground next to your thighs and lift your hips. Stay here for five breaths. Lower back to the ground, and remove your arms from between your legs.

2. *Trikonasana B*—Triangle Pose B

Trikonasana B is the first substantive twist in the Ashtanga Yoga method. Twisting can be an emotional journey into the center of the body. Trikonasana B expands the heart center, detoxifies the middle body, and stabilizes the legs.

Start in Samasthiti. Inhale as you step out to the right, leaving a distance slightly shorter than one leg-length between your feet. This distance is adjustable based on your height, leg length, and level of flexibility. Align your right heel with your left arch, square your hips, and fold forward. Suck in your lower belly as you glide your left hand across the center line of your body and place it on the floor along the outer edge of your right foot. If you cannot reach the floor comfortably, you can place your left hand either on your shin or on a block placed against the outer edge of your right foot. Align your left little finger with your right little toe. Inhale as you raise your right hand, lift your rib cage away from your hips, expand your chest, and twist along your spinal axis to fully enter Trikonasana B. Stay here for five breaths. Inhale as you come up and pivot your feet to repeat the pose on the left side. Return to Samasthiti after completing the left side.

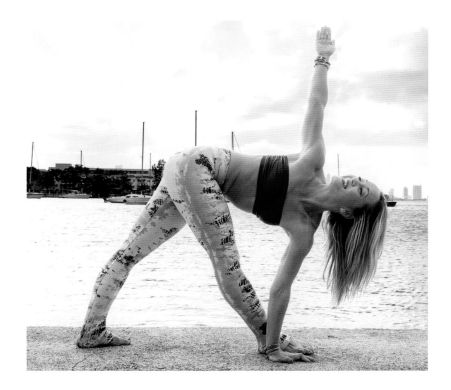

It can be very challenging to open your chest while maintaining balance. This expansion of the chest is one of the keys to opening the heart center and feeling your emotions.

3. *Anuvittasana*—Standing Backbend
There is perhaps no greater challenge between power and vulnerability in the practice than backbends. The tenacious valor of the warrior's strength is the foundation for the release into the openness of the deer's heart.

Step your feet hip-width apart, hands in prayer position, and plant your feet firmly on the ground. Engage your quadriceps, lift upward and inward with your pelvic floor, and draw your lower belly in. Expand your chest, and maximize the space between your ribs and hips and between each vertebra in your spine. Exhale as you send your hips forward, fold each of the joints of your spine backward, and drop your head back. Keep your hands in prayer position at the center of your chest. If you feel comfortable, extend your arms up and over the top of your head. Gaze over the top of your head toward the floor behind you. Stay here for at least five breaths. Then slowly return to standing by reversing the same instructions used to enter the pose. Send your hips forward, stack your rib cage on top of the hips, place your hands in prayer at the center of your chest, and inhale as you come back up.

Observe your emotions. Hanging over in a backbend often brings up fear, panic, anger, sadness, and a host of other emotions. Remain equanimous and repattern your neurological response to these difficult emotions. Bring your emotions up to the surface and accept them with the power of the breath, the pose, and the focal point.

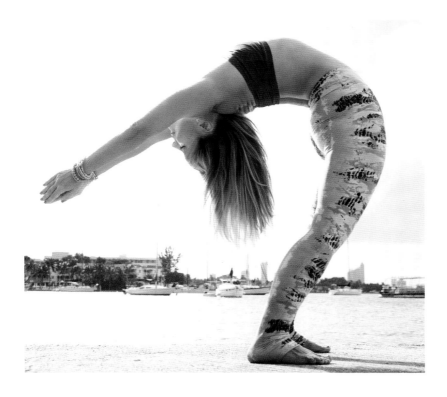

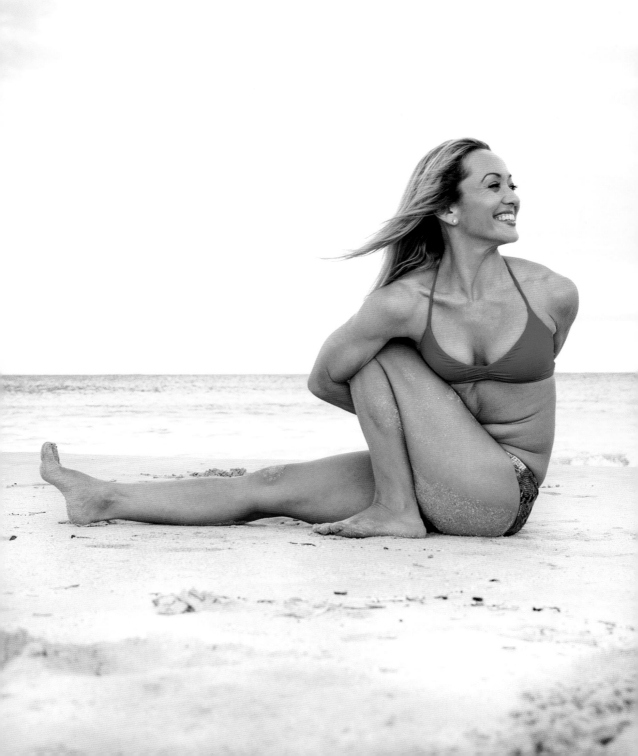

The Yogic State of Cleanliness
Saucha

Today's assignment, cleanliness, is a key principle in traditional yoga philosophy. Called *saucha* in Sanskrit, the practice of cleanliness is included in the eight-limbed path of Ashtanga Yoga under the moral and ethical observances (the niyamas). Yoga is a purification practice that reveals the light of the true self within through a systematic cleansing of the body, mind, and emotions.

In many ways, cleansing is kind of a modern trend. *Detoxification* is a catchword, not only for yoga classes but also for many holistic health remedies and treatments. However, according to the yoga tradition, saucha has a spiritual intention. Patanjali's Yoga Sutras state that practicing yogic cleanliness leads to a state called *jugupsa*, which is often translated as "distaste for the material state of embodiment." Some people mistakenly associate this with body hatred, but it is far from that. Saucha is a spiritual principle of purity that teaches you how to love and honor your body, mind, and environment. Jugupsa is perhaps better understood as the humble admission that we can never fully control or tame the material world. By devoting your efforts to purification, you may sometimes feel overwhelmed with the constant work necessary to keep all the aspects of the material world in a state of cleanliness. Just tending to household chores requires a lot of mindfulness and action.

However, your physical environment is only one aspect of all that needs tending in the material world. Your body itself is part of the material world, and its constant need for both external and internal grooming and cleaning presents almost a full-time job. The mind and its realm of thoughts can be said to be part of the material world; that is, the mind tends to think thoughts rooted in the material rather than the spiritual world. As such, the mind itself needs cleaning. While the task of cleaning the body, mind, and world can be daunting, the positive effect of jugupsa is that it helps us further appreciate and identify with yoga's spiritual quest.

In my quest for saucha when I first started yoga, I took on a massive detox and changed my diet dramatically. I went from being an average American meat eater to embracing a totally raw vegan diet over the course of just a few months. To say that I got a little obsessed would be an understatement! I also went on a series of fasts, cleanses, and flushes to get rid of toxins that many people in the yoga community explained were buried in my body. While I have been a vegetarian for almost twenty years, respect and truly love many foods from the raw vegan diet, and still engage in periodic fasting, the extremity with which I jumped into this process was simply not healthy for me. Instead of loving my body, I was punishing it. Saucha is never meant to be punitive.

Diet is a personal exercise in both ethics and health. The yogic practice of saucha is about balance and seeks to create health in the body, mind, and environment, while encouraging us to yearn for the spiritual truth of the inner self. Any path that focuses too strictly and exclusively on the body is a dead end. Yoga seeks to redefine the mind's point of awareness with the spirit; only when you see your natural inner purity is the state of saucha really possible. Certainly foods, thoughts, and actions can lead to further identification with the material world and enmesh you more deeply in the cycle of sensory pleasure and pain. Food and lifestyle choices make a difference in the health of your body and in the general state of the world around you, in both your home and your community.

The yogi's commitment to saucha is a testing point for all actions and choices that each practitioner must personally make. To say that you can eat whatever you want because you are internally pure is a delusion. To say that you are made whole and pure by what you eat is equally deluded. Instead, food choices are merely a reflection of an inner state of resolution. The commitment to saucha also means that you cannot hide from the impact that your actions have on the world. Cleanliness is both a ritual of personal hygiene and a social responsibility. It makes no sense to eat a pure diet while engaging in practices that pollute the earth. Yet saucha is not meant to perfect the spirit through rules and dogmas enacted in the flesh. Saucha is a spiritual practice that encourages you to root the true point of self-identification in the eternality of the spirit within. While it may be easier to take on strict dogmas in the effort toward purification and cleanliness, saucha is more an inner state of unconditional love than it is a set or series of rules to follow. You have to find out for yourself what that path is and then walk it with integrity.

The spiritual heart is always pure. There is a seat of sacredness deep within you that cannot be defiled by any action. Grace and beauty are within you. Not one soul lacks the spark of brilliance. But many of us turn away from the light we have within. We believe the lies our weakness and doubt tell us, that we are unworthy of love. But none of that is true. The purity of your spirit is all the grace you need. You don't need to struggle and try to be someone else. You just need to show up and be 100 percent, purely, cleanly yourself.

1. Practice saucha of thought. Cleanse your thoughts—what you think reflects your intention in life. A great way to purify your thoughts is to watch what you say and speak only life-affirming words (toward yourself and others) that infuse your world with peace and love. Note any self-directed negative comments that you make under your breath. Never punish or berate yourself. Ask yourself if you believe all your thoughts to be true. If so, ask which thoughts may actually be opinions and not absolutely true. Question your thoughts and clean out your mind.

2. Practice saucha of body. Your regular yoga practice cleanses your body. Try the series of poses in the practice section. Eat healthful and nourishing food today. Do a juice fast if you feel you need a little extra cleanse, or just do a minicleanse by eliminating one type of food (like dairy, wheat, or meat) from your diet for a day as an experiment. Consider trying a vegetarian or vegan diet one day a week for a year. Write about it in your journal and see how you feel.

3. Practice saucha of the world. We all have a space in our home or know a place that we frequent that could use a little attention. Go find that neglected closet and clean it out, empty old items out of the fridge and pantry, sweep the floor. When you step outside your home, pick up a stray piece of trash on the street. Do something positive for the earth!

PRACTICE

1. *Marichyasana C*—Pose Dedicated to Sage Marichi C

Twisting is one of the most powerful agents of inner cleansing, and this pose is a great place to learn the basics of twisting. Twisting poses wash and fold the body from the inside out and encourage a deeper inner awareness of the body.

Start in Dandasana (Staff Pose) and draw your left knee in toward your chest. Allow a gentle internal rotation of the left hip joint so that your left knee slides toward your left armpit. Place your left foot flat on the ground. Keep both sitting bones firmly planted on the ground. Draw your lower belly in deeply, hollow out your pelvic bowl, and begin leaning to the left. Fold your torso around your left thigh, and draw your ribs in to twist from the center. Exhale as you wrap your right elbow around your left shin. Complete the pose by reaching your left hand up behind your back and binding your hands above your right hip. If you cannot bind your hands, drop your right shoulder around the left thigh, place your right hand or fingertips on the ground, extend your left arm toward the floor in back of you for support, and focus on the signal twist. Look over your left shoulder. Hold the pose for at least five breaths and then return to Dandasana. Repeat on the right side.

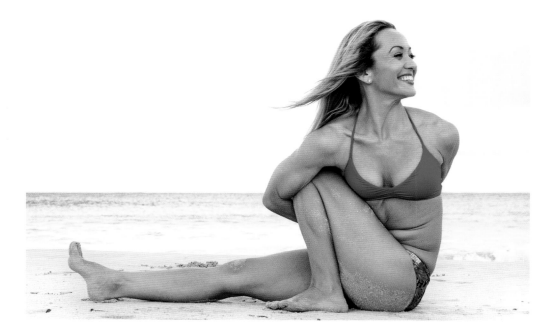

2. *Padangusthasana*—Hand-to-Big-Toe Pose

Forward folds encourage a cleansing of the digestive system and create a sense of emptiness in the pelvic bowl. Padangusthasana is a deep forward fold that brings you face-to-face with the need to cleanse your body.

Start in Samasthiti and step your feet hip-width apart. Send your pubic bone back and up to facilitate folding through the hip joints. Avoid rounding your back. Fold forward and wrap your fingers around your big toes. Inhale, lifting your chest while lengthening your spine. Exhale as you fold farther into the space you create deep within the inner body. If you cannot grab your toes with your legs straight, bend your knees slightly so you can wrap your fingers firmly around your toes and then attempt to straighten your legs. Maintain a sense of emptiness in your pelvic bowl. Stay here for five breaths. Inhale, straighten your arms, and gently look up. Exhale, firm your pelvic floor, and rise back to Samasthiti.

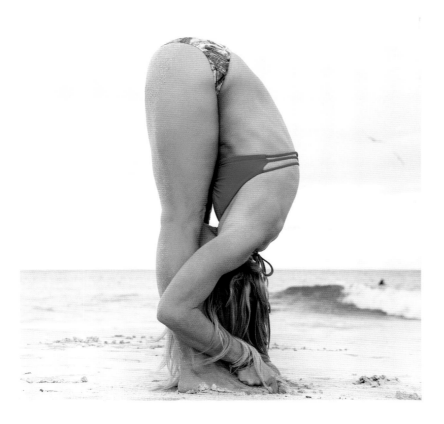

3. *Bakasana*—Crane Pose

Strength is a big part of inner cleansing. It is often the arm balances that cultivate the inner fire and heat of purification. Bakasana relies on the emptiness created in deep forward folds combined with the activation of inner fire.

Start off in a squatting position and place your knees in your armpits. Keep your arms as straight as possible. If you need to bend your elbows, avoid splaying your arms out to the side. Engage your pelvic floor, firm your lower abdominal muscles, draw your lower ribs in, and send your weight forward into the stability of your shoulders. Firm your shoulder girdle, and send your hips back and up. Gaze toward your nose. Press your knees forward, draw your feet up toward your hips, grip your fingertips into the floor, and lift up into Bakasana. If you cannot lift up into the full pose, then stop when you lean your weight forward and lift one foot at a time, alternating until you feel strong enough to lift both feet. Stay here for five breaths. Exhale and return to a squatting position. Repeat up to three times.

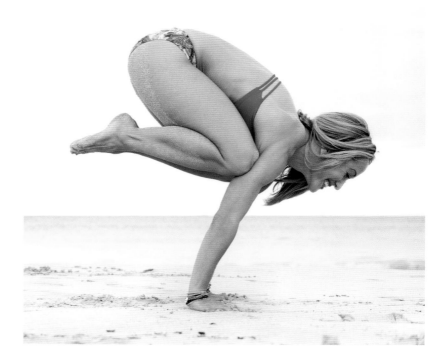

4. Mayurasana—Peacock Pose

This powerful arm balance is probably the most traditionally cleansing pose in the yoga practice. Mayurasana is said to strengthen the stomach and digestive system, making it immune to toxins. Peacocks are famous for being able to consume normally poisonous animals as part of their diet with no harmful effects.

Start off in a kneeling position. Turn your hands backward so that your fingers point toward your toes. Align your little fingers and elbows. Bend your elbows and place them in the center of your abdomen at the solar plexus. Stabilize your shoulder girdle, firm your abdominal muscles, and send your body weight forward as you lift your legs to enter Mayurasana. Avoid arching your back; instead, use the strength of the front of your body to enter and stabilize the pose.

This pose took me years to integrate fully, so be patient. If you can't lift both legs, then lift one foot at a time and alternate until you feel strong enough to lift both feet. Stay here for five breaths. Repeat up to three times. To exit Mayurasana, simply place your feet on the ground, bend your knees, and remove your hands.

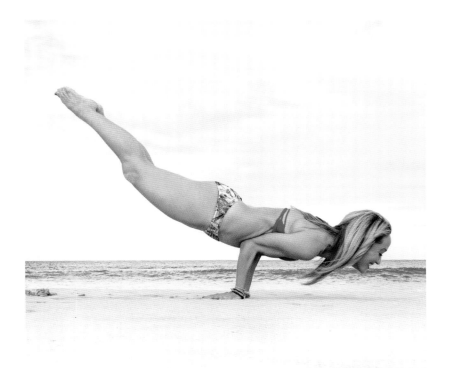

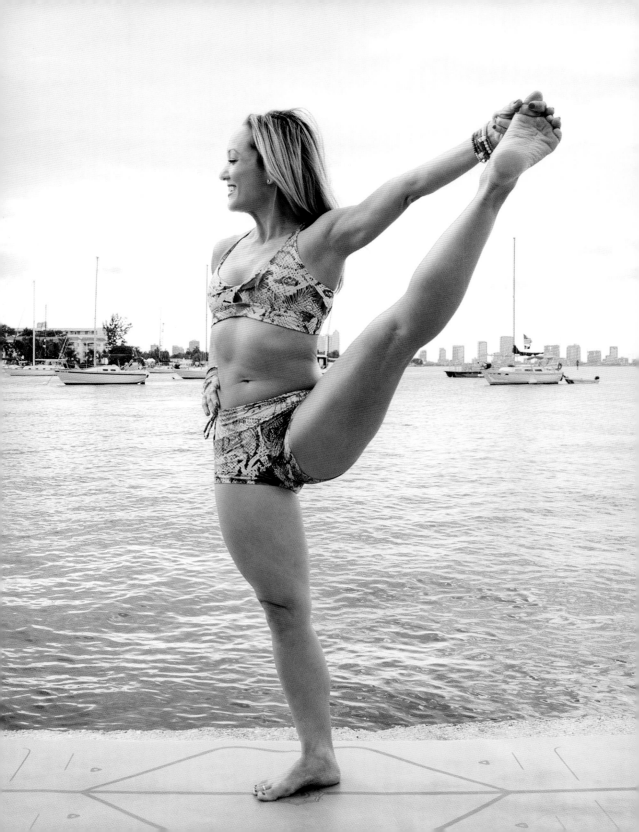

Choose to Be Content
Santosha

When someone asks you how you are, is your automatic response "Busy"? Busyness is addictive. It has an inertia that seems to draw more and more activity into its swirling vortex. It can feel impossible to stop! It is a mild mania where the perpetual running means you stay so busy that you don't have to feel anything. Yoga is a path that runs counter to this busy state of mind—and it helps you start to recognize the clutter in your mental and emotional world.

One of the most powerful vrittis in modern life is the heightened state of arousal caused by our perpetual busyness, our obsessive focus on reaching the next big milestone. This constant be-more, do-more attitude ensures that your nervous system operates in a jacked-up state that can come close to panic. So many of us are addicted to the feeling of stress that the idea of relaxing, dialing it down, and tuning in to the inner world seems impossible. To the stress-addicted mind, nothing is ever good enough; we are never satisfied. Instead, we are caught in a cyclical state of self-induced unhappiness and discontent. The whirl-wind of a busy lifestyle feels like we are caught in the wheel of samsara, sometimes understood as the wheel of time that spins a web of illusion based on the creation of a false self—that is, the ego.

Samsara busyness happens when your actions are rooted in the ego's sense of "me" and "mine," pleasure and pain, attachment and aversion. The ego searches for permanent happiness and a stable point on the ever-changing wheel of samsara, but it does not find them. Samsara is the decision to enter the cosmic rat race in an attempt to reach some unknown destination of future promised success. But just under the surface of all that busyness is one big, busy mess! Emotions you'd rather not feel, like sadness, depression, anger, anxiety, self-pity, and fear, lurk in the subconscious mind. Physical issues like chronic pain, persistent injuries, sickness, or other ailments that require attention but fall last on the busy person's priorities list are one of the many ways the body internalizes unprocessed stress. Most often, the ego runs because it is afraid to face the simple truths of pain and suffering that are held within a wounded heart.

No matter how fast your world spins or how busy you really are, this is your life and you have a choice. All you have to do is stop long enough to breathe through your emotional armor and be strong enough to face whatever you are running from.

Most busyness operates from a sense of emptiness; there is a void inside that drives you to throw yourself into activities and achievements to prove you are "worthy." I know this state all too well. There were times when I felt I needed to prove my worth as a human being through my achievements and by how hard I worked on certain asanas. Then, when my father's health took a drastic turn for the worse and I faced difficulties in my marriage, my first inclination was to work more and throw myself into a breakneck schedule that never stopped. Although the wheels of my life were turning at full speed, they were doomed to crash because they were founded on the perspective of what I lacked. Thankfully, my yoga path showed me the way out of my own busy mess.

Traditional yoga philosophy has the antidote to modern busyness. It posits that only by learning how to accept yourself exactly as you are, in the fullness and completeness of your being, will you find true, lasting peace and joy. The contentment that comes from this total self-acceptance is called *santosha*. Santosha is the happiness that comes from tuning in to the eternal place of truth within you, the place where you already have everything you need, where all is good and complete, and where you have access to all the love in the universe. This is actually the only place that is real. Santosha is a strong, equanimous mind that is free of insecurity, full and whole, resting in the wisdom of a full heart and a clear mind. Santosha is contained within the niyamas, the second of the eight limbs of Ashtanga Yoga aimed at personal observances according to the yogic path.

There will always be something to distract your mind in the sea of busyness. There will always be another email to answer; another promotion to work for; a fancier car, a fatter bank account, or a bigger house to get. Recognize these for what they are—distractions that take you just far enough off course to get lost and unfocused, making you confused about what really matters. Practicing the state of mind known as santosha will give you the strength to keep yourself dedicated to the spiritual intention of life. Rather than one specific practice, santosha is a paradigm shift that affects every action you take. It's like updating the operating system of your mind and recalibrating the metrics of success. The goal of every day in the yoga life is to love more; to stay true to the spiritual heart; and to honor, respect, and cherish one another in love. The yogi is ever vigilant against the large and small grievances that show up in an overly busy life. If left unchecked, these often unspoken thoughts plant the seeds of bitterness, jealousy, or animosity toward other people (or toward oneself).

It may surprise you to know that I never felt particularly good at yoga practice. In fact, I felt so clumsy that I would often leave my mat with a sense of defeat. After nearly twenty years of practice, I still feel uncoordinated whenever I flail around trying a new pose. The difference between then and now is that I'm no longer bothered by it. That is the power of the santosha attitude. I'm perfectly content to fall on my butt now. I actually do it with a smile and a laugh, whereas before it would make me mad and unhappy. Contentment happens when you understand your true nature; then every action is a reflection of the wholeness within you. Whenever you feel yourself veering off course, pause, check yourself, and redirect your mind back to the deeper purpose of your life. Busyness is replaced with beingness if you decide to choose santosha.

HOMEWORK **1. Practice santosha in thought.** Practice cultivating an equanimous mind. Next time you have an experience that could easily register as "good" or "bad," drop the story line and simply observe what is, without any judgment. Focus on your breath for ten counts, and observe the breath in its natural state. Let inhalation be inhalation; let exhalation be exhalation. Just observe the experience as it naturally unfolds and be content with it as it is. Refrain from making any value judgments or telling any stories about what is happening. Say the words, "What is simply is," and let the sensations be.

2. Practice santosha in your world. Notice the areas in your daily life about which you habitually complain—like the weather, politics, or traffic. When you are about to complain, check yourself. Instead of lapsing into annoyance, first simply observe what is and then practice accepting what is. Make peace with your world. Check back in through-out the day to reconfirm your commitment to santosha. If you are in a traffic jam, simply observe, *I am in a traffic jam*. Make it neither good nor bad. Let it be as it is. Refrain from telling any positive or negative stories about your current situation. Just be.

3. Remember "I am enough." Focus your attention on your heart. See yourself as filled with light, and let that inner light nourish your soul and fill your whole body, like an overflowing fountain. Say the words "I am enough."

PRACTICE **1.** *Utkatasana*—Chair Pose

This pose allows you to make peace with difficulty and build spiritual endurance. Start in Samasthiti at the front of your mat, with the bases of your big toes together and a small space between your heels. Sink into your hip joints as you bend your knees deeply. Draw your inner thighs toward each other while firming your quadriceps. Suck your lower belly in to support your spine and lower back. Lift your rib cage and torso while maintaining the deep flexion in your hips. Straighten your arms up toward the ceiling and press your palms together. Gaze up

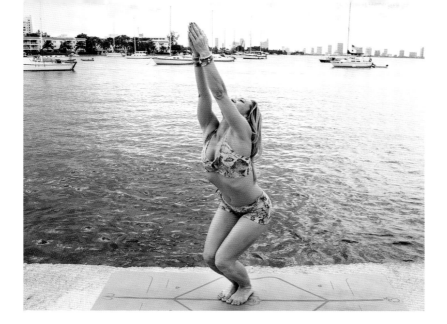

at your thumbs to fully enter Utkatasana. Stay here for five breaths, then return to Samasthiti.

Your thighs may burn throughout this pose. Practice remaining equanimous, and be content with the small amount of discomfort that inevitably arises in your thighs. Observe, *My thighs are on fire*, and stay in the pose.

2. *Utthita Hasta Padangusthasana*— Extended Hand-to-Big-Toe Pose

As in any balancing pose, the effort of attaining balance often involves a lot of falling. This process will challenge your santosha state of mind.

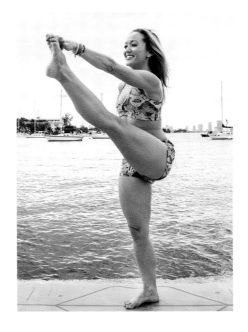

Start in Samasthiti. Inhale as you bend your left knee, raise your leg, and wrap your fingers around your left big toe. Once you find your balance, straighten your left leg out and up by drawing backward with your left hip. If you can successfully straighten your leg, suck your belly in and exhale to fold forward, aligning your sternum with your knee. If you cannot straighten your leg, then do not fold forward; simply remain standing and work on your balance. Stay here for five breaths.

Inhale to lift your torso while stabilizing the pose with the strength of your pelvic floor. Exhale as you externally rotate your left hip joint and bring your leg out to the side. Look toward the right. Again, if you cannot straighten your leg yet, simply hold your big toe with your knee bent. Stay here for five breaths. Inhale, bring your left leg back to center, and stabilize the pose. Exhale and fold forward, bringing your sternum down toward your knee and your hip back. Inhale as you come back up, keeping your leg raised; place your hands on your waist and balance. Hold the balance for five breaths. Return to Samasthiti. Repeat on the right side.

Utthita Hasta Padangusthasana often brings up frustration and impatience because it demands a high level of both balance and flexibility. Practice santosha by accepting wherever you are in the pose without needing to go any further. If you fall or lose your balance, remain equanimous, observe that you have fallen or lost your balance, and try again.

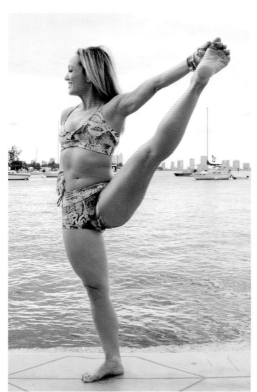
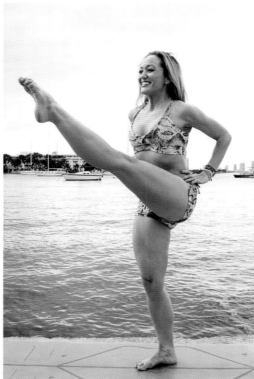

3. *Bhujapidasana*—Shoulder Pressing Pose

Begin in Adho Mukha Svanasana (Downward-Facing Dog Pose). Inhale as you jump or step forward, placing your feet outside your hands. Bend your elbows and your knees slightly to settle your thighs onto the shelves of your upper arms. Activate and lift up with your pelvic floor. Lift your feet off the ground, wrap your lower legs around your arms, and cross your ankles in front of you. If you cannot cross your ankles easily, do not proceed to the full expression of the pose. Instead, simply work to your limit and practice santosha.

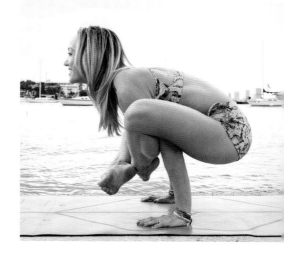

Exhale as you pivot forward, placing your head or chin on the ground while sliding your feet back behind your hands. Stay here for five breaths. Inhale, lift your head, and slide your feet forward again. Exhale, release your ankles, slide your feet back around the outside of your arms, and jump back to Chaturanga Dandasana.

Many students will feel a sense of failure when they try this pose. It is common for your butt to sink toward the ground and slide back and down. Each time you fall back, observe that you have fallen back and accept where you are without feeling a need to rush the process.

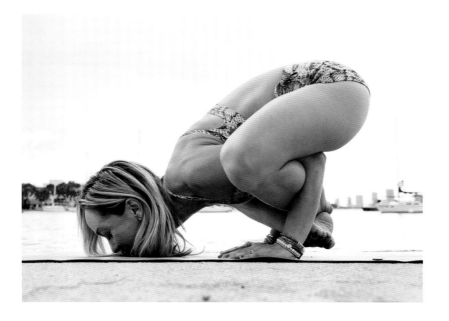

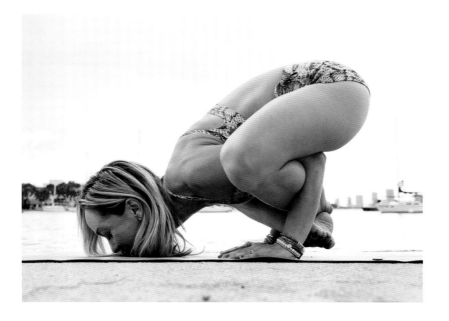

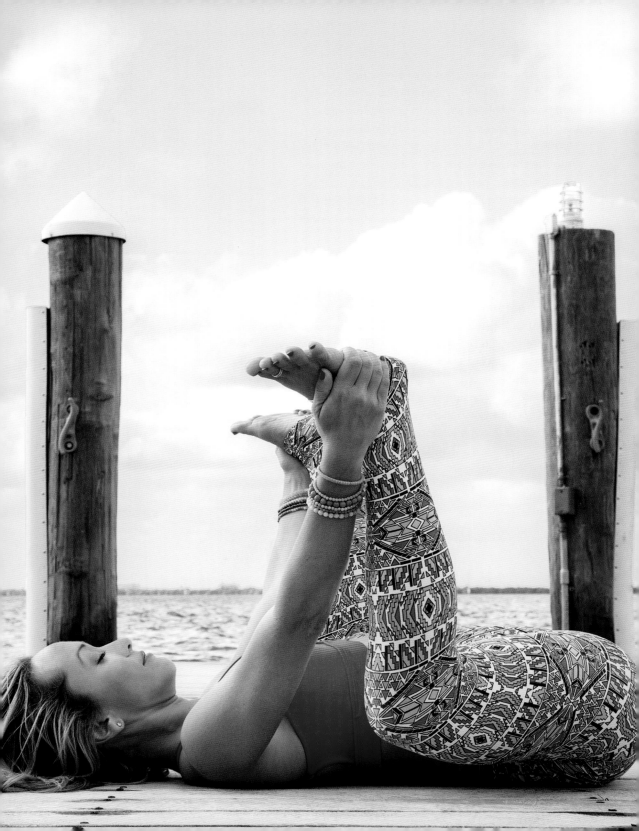

Nonviolence
Ahimsa

oga breaks through the glossy layers of the outer self to reveal the tender, aching heart of compassion and empathy that each of us has within. Every time you suffer in yoga, your heart expands and grows bigger. By becoming brave enough to feel everything, you are making yourself strong enough to take on the vow of ahimsa (nonviolence). Shri K. Pattabhi Jois always waited for students to ask about the moral and ethical principles of yogic living before talking about these tenets. It was as though he knew that until the heart is made ready by the rigors of practice, it serves no purpose to give students a new dogma to replace whatever rules and guidelines they already adhere to.

Today's yogi assignment is ahimsa. In Patanjali's Yoga Sutras, ahimsa is the first of the moral and ethical principles for yogic living. It is the "bowl" that holds the other eight limbs and makes yoga practice possible. *Himsa* is the Sanskrit word for "violence," and *ahimsa* is translated as "nonviolence." But it could be argued that ahimsa is not only nonviolence but the opposite of violence: compassion, mercy, peace, and love. Patanjali further presents ahimsa as the great vow, called *mahavrtam* in Sanskrit. This great vow is not a legalistic dogma to be judged by others but the sincerity of the yoga practitioner's heart. Students can take on some aspects of ahimsa—like veganism or environmentalism—but if they do so judgmentally and without compassion, their practice misses the mark completely. Violence takes many forms, and the first step toward a more peaceful life is to recognize the violence that we either have been subject to or have subjected others to in our lives. Often that violence appears as judgment toward or a lack of compassion for ourselves and others.

The best yogi acts as a force of healing in the world. Start your journey by ending violence within your own life. Begin by cultivating an attitude of acceptance, tolerance, and compassion for yourself. Make peace with yourself, your body, your successes, and your failures. Commit no acts of self-directed negativity in speech, thought, or deed. Don't beat yourself up when you practice. Embrace your body. Don't try to mold it into someone else's shape—the perfect body for practice is the one you have. I wasted too many years of my life hating my body. Self-directed hatred eats away at your self-worth and leaves a shell of unhappiness that is far more damaging than anything you eat or don't eat. Instead, treat your body as a sacred space of worship and speak only life-affirming words to yourself. The state of ahimsa must begin with the deep resolution of self-love.

Once you have started to build a peaceful relationship with yourself, turn your attention to the world around you. Maintain the commitment to ahimsa in your speech, thoughts, and actions when interacting with people throughout your day. Pay careful attention to your tone of voice when speaking with your partner, friends, and family members. At the very least, seek to do no harm. Notice any negative or violent thoughts, and take responsibility for them. Refrain from taking any action rooted in negativity.

Next, turn your attention to the impact your actions make on the world at large. You may feel an overwhelming desire to volunteer for a social mission, foster stray animals, or lobby political leaders for changes you want to see in the world.

You may find, as I did, that the choice to switch to a plant-based diet just feels right. No one ever told me that I should be vegetarian or vegan, and I am not telling you that you should follow this path. My practice led me to question the health of my diet. Then I read a book about the ethical implications of large-scale, commercialized animal husbandry and the environmental impact of livestock. I was overwhelmed with compassion for the animals and the earth, and I knew that the choice to switch to a plant-based diet was right for me. If you asked Shri K. Pattabhi Jois about the yoga diet, he would always respond with the same answer: "simple vegetarian food." But he never forced anyone to make that change.

While ahimsa is usually associated with the moral and ethical choice to follow a vegetarian or vegan diet, it is far more than that. Some of the angriest people I've ever met have been vegetarians, and some of the most peaceful people I've known have eaten meat. Living the yogi's life is not about creating a dogma and then judging others when they fail to live up to it. We all fail to follow ahimsa perfectly. Every harsh word or thought, every seed of bitterness or jealousy, every piece of nonrecyclable plastic, every use of nuclear power, and every full gas tank could be seen as a violation of ahimsa. I believe in yoga, but truly, I believe in you. A generation of yogis can change the world! Only when cultural values change on a large scale will we see the kind of global change that can heal the earth.

Goodness is action. Your heart is always evident in your actions. You can say you value something, but it is how you truly spend your time that tells the story of what you value. The commitment to ahimsa is a living promise between your spirit and the world. Devote yourself to the principle of ahimsa and truly live the yogi's life. Don't let anyone else tell you what it means to be a yogi; follow your heart. Let your actions tell the story of your heart's commitment to make your world a more peaceful place.

1. Practice ahimsa in speech and thought. Make a commitment to speak only life-affirming words and think positive thoughts about yourself and your world for one full day. Catch yourself before saying anything negative. Do not lie and refrain from any mean-spirited dialogue, which means no rants, no anonymous negative comments on social media, no arguments of any type.

2. Consider an ahimsa diet. Take a conscious look at your dietary choices and the impact they have on the world. If you are a meat eater, reflect on the source of your meat and what the animal went through to become the piece of flesh in your meal. If you are a vegetarian, consider if the sources of your animal products such as dairy are indeed ethical sources. If you are a vegan, think about the means of production and agricultural processes that created the food you eat. Commit to making one meal a day that involves the least amount of violence to the world possible.

3. Practice self-healing. Our greatest source of violence may be ourselves. We internalize negativity or punish ourselves harshly for perceived shortcomings and failures. For one day, commit to engaging in only positive inner dialogue and a ritual of self-affirmation. Moment to moment, reflect on all the things you did well and forgive yourself for any mistakes you made. Each time you find yourself doubting or judging yourself, stop and turn the thought around. Instead of focusing on some part of your body that you don't like, focus on a part that you do like. If you find it impossible to speak positive words to yourself, then simply refrain from negative inner dialogue.

4. Practice world healing. The earth is in need of our commitment to live a more peaceful life. Evaluate each of your actions and its impact on the environment from a resources and pollution perspective. Are there changes you can make that will decrease the impact you have on the planet? Is there a cause that aligns with your passion toward which you can dedicate time and energy?

PRACTICE

1. *Ananda Balasana*—Happy Baby Pose

Ananda Balasana offers you a chance to make peace with your hips and ultimately yourself.

Start off in a supine position. Inhale as you lift your legs, bend your knees, and fold your thighs in toward your torso. Spread your thighs slightly wider than your torso, and keep your lower legs vertical. Reach up to hold on to the outer edges of your feet. Keep your sacrum as close to the ground as possible and lift it only as much as necessary to make the contact between your hands and feet. Gaze up toward the ceiling or close your eyes. Keep your lower belly drawn in to support your lower back. Take at least five breaths. Return slowly to a supine position.

Once you reach a comfortable state, settle your sacrum down into the ground while maintaining the connection between your hands and feet. Notice any negative thoughts that arise, perhaps about your body size or shape or any limitation in your hips. Cultivate a peaceful and restorative attitude toward your body.

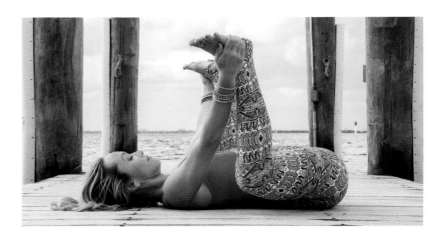

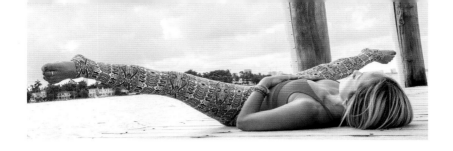

2. Supta Samakonasana—Reclining Straddle Pose

This is a restorative pose that helps you cultivate a peaceful attitude of self-acceptance.

Start off in a supine position. Inhale as you lift your legs, keeping them together. Settle your sacrum on the ground and suck in your lower belly. Exhale as you open your legs to release and stretch your inner thighs. Keep your quadriceps engaged and actively reach outward through both legs. Point your toes and avoid being passive. Stay here for ten breaths. Slowly inhale as you bring your legs back together. Exhale as you lower them back to the ground.

Cultivate a peaceful and accepting attitude. Practice not forcing your body into any pose or demanding that it go too deep. Just be exactly where you are and accept yourself.

3. Supta Matsyendrasana—Supine Spinal Twist

This simple pose is the perfect place to practice self-healing. Start off in a supine position. Inhale as you bring your right knee in toward your chest. Hold on to your right knee with your left hand. Exhale as you twist across the center line and reach your right knee toward the ground on your left side. Stabilize your left leg and keep it straight. Extend your right arm out to the side in line with your shoulders. Draw your subnavel in and activate your pelvic floor. Turn your head and look toward the right. Stay here for five to ten breaths, then return to center and repeat on the left side.

Find the inner space of peace and acceptance. Let go of any self-directed negativity and just be.

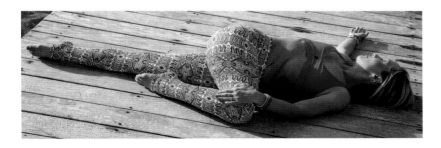

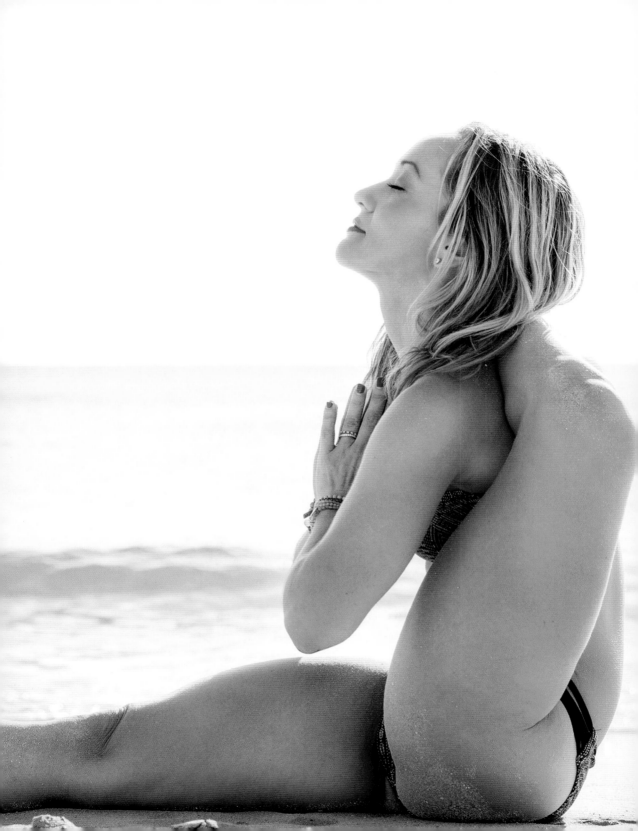

am not a naturally patient person. The moment I have a new idea, I want it to have already happened! By nature, I focus on the result, not the process. So when I was first learning the many challenging advanced poses in Ashtanga Yoga, I came across several new obstacles that did not respond to my desire for immediate results. I used to psych myself up each day by saying, "Today is my day!" One day, in a mad rush to master one of the more difficult poses, I repeated that phrase fifteen times. Suffice it to say that approach only left me feeling exhausted and defeated. Over nearly twenty years of practice, I have learned how to be patient with myself, my body, and my world, and you can too.

When I traveled to Mysore, India, for the first time, I met my teachers, Shri K. Pattabhi Jois and R. Sharath Jois. After eight months of practice, I was feeling impatient about the arrival of the lofty goal of samadhi, or ultimate peace. When I questioned the Ashtanga Yoga method, Shri K. Pattabhi Jois let me know that the yoga path is a very long one; I would have to be patient, work consistently, and surrender to and have faith in myself and the method. I am so thankful I did. One of the most humbling things about the practice is that you do not get to decide when and where things happen. Each pose unfolds at its own pace, and the body takes its own time. Just like a flower has its own time to sprout, blossom, bloom, and maybe even bear fruit, so too does your body have its own time to open, release, strengthen, and surrender. The more you push and force, the less likely it is that your body will open and progress.

Today's yogi assignment is patience, defined in the Bhagavad Gita as *kshanti*, or the cultivation of patient self-control, restraint, and tolerance. Patience is one of the qualities of a spiritual warrior. Yoga is a path of self-knowledge, and the poses are mirrors of the inner world. How you approach your practice is a microcosm of how you approach your life. By learning how to be patient when you face a yoga pose that brings up anxiety, frustration, irritation, depression, and even anger, you learn how to be patient when life situations trigger those same emotions. There is an infinite number of annoying situations in life—flight delays, traffic jams, bad cups of coffee, snide remarks, smelly bathrooms—the list is truly endless. The more something bothers you, the easier it is to react harshly and let the apparent urgency of your personal suffering be the driver of your life. It is harder to pause, reflect, and breathe. The ability to bear things that are uncomfortable requires great spiritual strength. Imagine that the next time you are about to lose your temper with someone you love, you decide instead to take ten deep breaths. Imagine that instead of honking your horn at a traffic jam when you are already late for work, you decide to engage your pelvic floor and tune in to the inner body. Imagine that the next time your barista makes you a bad cup of coffee or gets your order wrong, you respond with an understanding smile. Your world will be more peaceful.

Some poses have taken me my entire yoga career to master, and even more still remain elusive. In many ways, I am still the same person I was when I first started my practice. I meet these difficult poses on my mat every day and work on getting stronger physically, emotionally, and spiritually. When I look at my practice in this way, I no longer judge myself for my inability to perform certain asanas. Instead, I respond to my body and my practice with patience and understanding because I am developing my inner self. Patience is the antidote to the craving for instant gratification and for judging your self-worth by the yardstick of external accomplishment.

Cultivating kshanti may only be possible by surrendering to faith in something bigger than you—God, the true light of the world, however you want to think about the presence of a Higher Power in the universe. Without faith, it is hard to grasp the magnificence of every moment in your life. You are here for a reason, and everything is unfolding exactly as it should. That reason may not always be evident to you, but if you trust that you are exactly where you need to be at this moment in time, then you will have the patience to attain what you want. Infinite patience often brings immediate results, because it brings with it an attitude of love and acceptance. Patience is the decision to wait for the promise of unseen things yet to come. It is the choice to wait out adversity, no matter how long it takes, with full faith. In other words, it is the long, winding road of the spiritual path.

1. Be patient about practice. Is there a yoga pose about which you feel impatient and judge yourself harshly for not attaining yet? Cultivate a patient and accepting attitude toward your body and yourself.

2. Don't worry, be patient. Is there a situation in your life that is clearly beyond your control, but you cannot help worrying about it? Is there a person in your life who just drives you nuts? Meditate for five to twenty minutes and ask for the burden of worry to be lifted from your heart. Cultivate a patient attitude about this situation, and ask to be granted understanding.

3. Use patient thinking. Reframe your point of attention toward the journey rather than the destination. Instead of focusing on the goal, change your point of attention to enjoying the process. Think of three things you appreciate about the process of where you are in your life or your yoga practice. Get lost in the details of the journey, then let time slow down.

1. *Eka Pada Sirsasana*—Foot-behind-the-Head Pose

PRACTICE

Just thinking about putting your leg behind your head can cause anxiety and frustration. Some students work on opening their hips consistently for more than a decade with little physical result. Regardless of where you are in your practice, take time to approach difficult poses like Eka Pada Sirsasana to cultivate a patient heart.

Start in a seated position with your legs straight. Inhale and externally rotate your left hip, dropping your knee out to the side. Hold your left foot with both hands, and drop your left shoulder forward. Slide your shinbone around the left shoulder, moving your foot behind your head. Release your left hand and use your right hand to adjust your left foot. Stabilize your pelvic floor, place your hands in prayer position at the center of your sternum, and look up to lock your leg in place. Exhale as you fold forward, aligning your sternum with your right knee.

PATIENCE KSHANTI

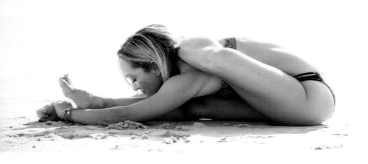

Wrap your hands around your right foot and gaze toward your right toes. Stay here for five breaths.

Inhale as you come up, then exhale as you place your hands on the ground. Try to keep your leg behind your head as you lift up and allow it to slide off only as you jump back. Inhale and lift up; exhale and jump back to Chaturanga Dandasana. Inhale and come forward to Urdhva Mukha Svanasana (Upward-Facing Dog Pose); exhale and roll back to Adho Mukha Svanasana. Inhale, jump through, and repeat the entire sequence on the right side.

Do not be surprised if your leg goes nowhere near your head. Go as far as possible and do not force it. Practice patience.

2. *Vrschikasana*—Scorpion Handstand Pose

I chose particularly hard poses for this chapter because I want to emphasize the longevity of the practice and the commitment it requires over many years. This handstand took me five years of consistent practice before I started to have any measure of success. It is a pose that I still work on to this day.

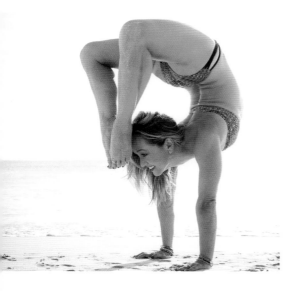

Start in a stable handstand. Extend your legs as far outward from your shoulders as possible, lengthening your spine as well as arching it, and lift your chest forward and up. Don't rush this part of the pose. Allow your knees to bend only after you have reached your maximum spinal extension. Exhale as you lift your head toward your feet and press firmly into the ground through your arms. Stay here for five breaths. Inhale as you return to handstand, and exhale as you come down into a simple forward fold.

Do not try to reach your feet to your head and force the pose or you will get a cramp in your hamstrings or toes and compress your back. If you do not have a stable handstand, then simply work on that. Be patient. Let it take as long as it takes.

3. *Natarajasana*—Lord of the Dance Pose

This pose evokes Lord Shiva, who appears as the cosmic dancer who seeks to destroy obstacles and illusions in the heart and prepares the way for a direct experience of God. Perhaps it's fitting then that Natarajasana often brings up frustration and impatience. Not only do you need flexibility in your hips, back, and shoulders, but you also need good balance and core strength. I cannot tell you how many times I have fallen out of this pose.

There are many different variations to the pose; the one illustrated here is one of the more advanced versions, but you can choose a more basic one. To achieve full Natarajasana only took me sixteen years! This pose is meant to be inspirational, not instructional. One key tip for all levels of Natarajasana is to lean forward, pivot into your hips, and send your navel down toward the ground. Avoid keeping your weight too "upright." And of course, be prepared to tumble out of the pose.

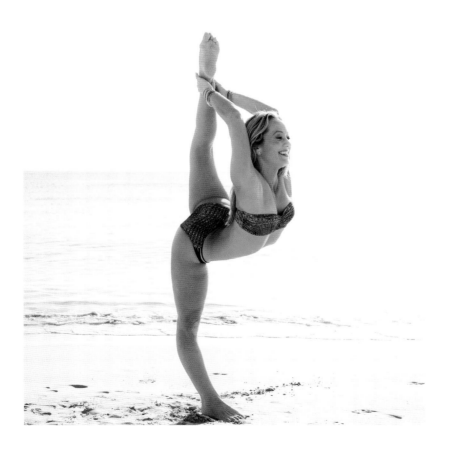

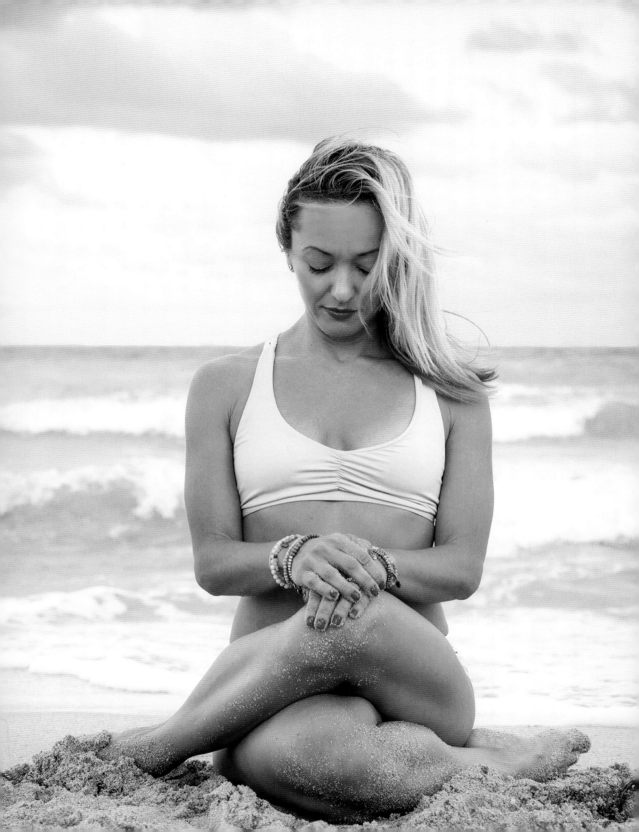

Selfless Service
Seva

hile it is easy to focus on perfecting your asana practice, the real yoga happens when you are strong enough within yourself to give more than you take in life. Yoga is giving back in the world, not just doing asanas. Today's yogi assignment is the yogic principle of service called *seva* in Sanskrit. Seva comprises acts of selfless service done with love and offered to the world out of the purity of your heart, with no expectation of recognition. Doing these acts, with no desire for reward, is a form of yoga.

Seva means to serve, attend to, worship, and pay homage to. There are at least two forms of service associated with seva—worship of God and service to humanity. The yogi is expected to engage in both forms of devotion. There are then three traditional categories of seva. The first is physical and consists of activities that engage your physical body. If you donate your time and effort to a cause, perform a service for someone, or give something away, this is a form of seva. Sometimes such activities are referred to as the dignity of physical labor. The second type of seva is mental and happens when you use your talents for the benefit of society rather than mere personal gain. An example of this type of service is when the brilliance of science is used to maximize social justice rather than capitalistic profits. The third type of seva is material and is often called *dana*; it includes offerings of money for charitable purposes or funds given to your guru or place of worship. Investing in others is an investment in your own happiness.

When I was twenty-two years old, I used all my personal savings and had financial support from my parents to travel to Mysore, India, for the first time to meet Shri K. Pattabhi Jois and R. Sharath Jois. It was a trip that changed my life and one that I was able to make only with the support I had. Not everyone has the same socioeconomic advantages that I did, so in collaboration with the charity Yogis Heart, I founded the Journey to India scholarship. This program awards one person annually a full scholarship to support one month's study at the

K. Pattabhi Jois Ashtanga Yoga Institute. Through an Instagram campaign, Yogis Heart and I raised more than $5,000 to cover the cost of airfare, housing, tuition, and living expenses. The scholarship is awarded based on merit and financial need through a board-reviewed application process, and it is one of the ways I choose to give back to the yoga community that has changed my life. What will your seva be?

Some people are afraid to give because they feel they have to save up their treasures for a rainy day. Others feel they have so little for themselves that it is impossible to give. The act of seva is a testament of faith. By giving freely—both of what you have and of what you feel you do not have—you make a statement of trust that you will receive all that you truly need. Not everyone has money, but we all have time and resources at our disposal. By cultivating a generous attitude and giving freely of what we do have, our hearts grow bigger, and we are fulfilled from the inside out. Let your whole life be a holy offering and a sacred prayer, let every breath be an act of reverence, let every action come from love. Be strong enough to be a force of healing in the world.

HOMEWORK
1. Perform random acts of kindness. Today go out into the world and ask where you can be of service, where a random act of kindness can make a positive difference in the world around you. Hold the door open for someone, hold the elevator, help someone carry groceries, pay for a cup of coffee for the person behind you in line.

2. Serve your friends and family. Look at the people in your inner circle, like your life partner, children, siblings, or parents, and ask yourself what you can do to serve them today. Are they stressed and in need of a little massage or a hug? Is there something you could take off their plate today just to make their lives easier?

3. Change your world. Volunteer and donate your time to a social mission that you believe will make your world a better place. Ask yourself what tugs at your heartstrings—animals, nature, children in need—and devote some part of your day to service. Find an organization through which you can give back in a meaningful way. You may choose to share your service on social media to raise awareness or keep it to yourself as a personal project.

1. *Visvamitrasana*—Visvamitra's Pose

This pose takes its name from the ancient sage Visvamitra, a king who renounced all his wealth after he gained powers through spiritual sacrifice and service. Visvamitra was known as a master of the disciplined practice of tapas. When practicing this powerful arm balance think of how you can be strong enough to give back to your world.

Start in Adho Mukha Svanasana. Inhale as you step your left foot forward and outside your left hand. Externally rotate your left hip joint and stack your left leg around your left shoulder. Keep your left knee bent. Inhale as you send your weight to the left side. Press down firmly on your left hand and come over into a left-side Utthita Chaturanga Dandasana (Plank Pose) while keeping your left leg tucked around your left shoulder. Plant your right foot into the ground. Exhale and firm your left shoulder and core. If you do not feel comfortable here, stop and do not proceed to the full expression of this pose. Inhale as you lift your right arm, straighten your left leg, and gaze up toward your right hand. Stay here for five breaths.

Exhale as you jump back to Chaturanga Dandasana. Inhale and come forward to Urdhva Mukha Svanasana, then exhale as you roll back to Adho Mukha Svanasana. Repeat on the left side.

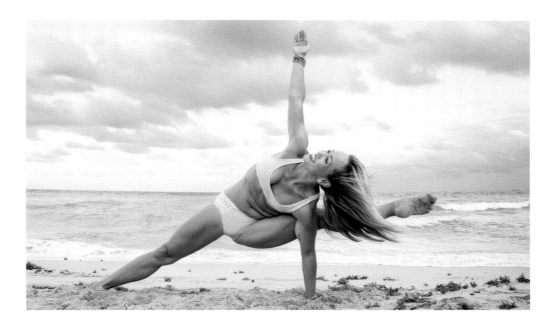

2. *Vatayanasana*—Horse Pose

The Sanskrit root of this word is *vatayana*, which can be translated into English as "horse" or "moving with the wind." Horses are significant animals in the Vedas; the animals appear as chariots that carry *devas* to the celestial abodes. The horse itself can be said to symbolize a powerful driving force in your life. When practicing Vatayanasana, think about channeling this inner power into contributing to your society.

Start in Samasthiti. Fold your left leg into Ardha Padmasana (Half Lotus). If you cannot do Half Lotus, then modify by kneeling on your left knee. Exhale as you bend your right leg and settle the top of your left knee on the ground. Place your right heel directly in front of your left knee. Place your hands on the ground to help you balance. Inhale and lift your torso. Thread your arms around each other, placing your left arm on top. Flatten your palms against each other, and lift your hands upward. Gaze toward your thumbs. Stay here for five breaths, then gently come down and return to Samasthiti. Repeat on the right side.

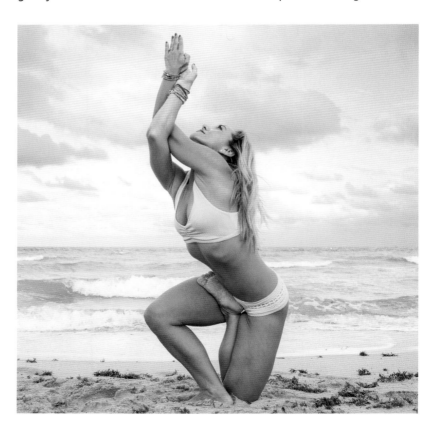

3. *Sukha Gomukhasana*—Relaxed Cow-Face Pose

The Sanskrit root of this asana name comes from the conjunction of the word for "cow" (*go*) and the word for "head" (*mukha*). The Sanskrit word *go* also means "light," so there may be a deeper meaning to the pose than merely mimicking the face of a cow. Cows themselves are considered sacred in India and serve a valuable purpose in society. The cow is portrayed as a gentle, kind creature that happily gives more than it takes. Cow's milk and products made from cows like ghee in traditional India are considered to be *sattvic* and healing for the body. The cow represents not only all living beings but also the earth itself, which continually provides sustenance for all its inhabitants. As such, cows are garlanded, honored, and given special status in Indian society. It must be noted that this veneration of cows is almost totally absent in the conventional dairy farming in most countries. While practicing Gomukhasana, reflect on the quality of gentleness, the respect for all living beings, and the goodness of soul required to truly give more than you take.

Start in a seated position with your legs straight. To enter the pose, fold your left thigh over your right, aligning your knees over each other and your feet on either side of your hips. Place your hands together over your left knee. Suck in your belly, gently arch your back, and gaze at the tip of your nose. Stay here for five breaths, then repeat on the right side.

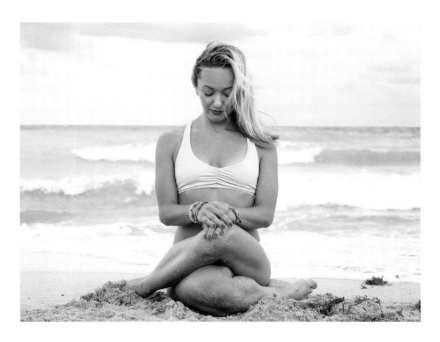

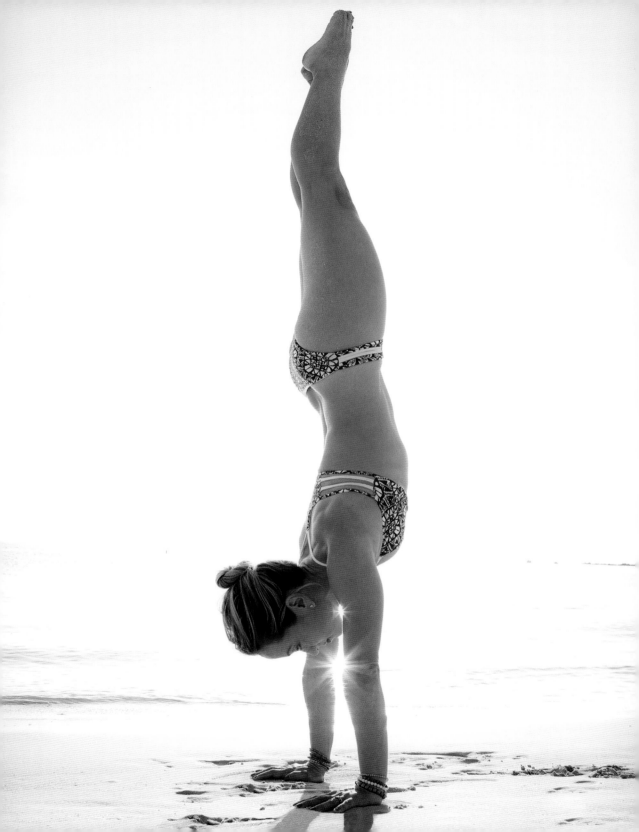

Day 8 | The Equanimous Mind
Upekshanam

A yogi is defined by more than just the ability to twist his or her body into various pretzel shapes; a yogi is someone who has the quality of mind to remain steady and balanced in the midst of life's inevitable ups and downs. Today's yogi assignment is *upekshanam* (equanimity). The equanimous mind is characterized by mental calmness, composure, and an even temper, especially in the face of difficult situations. Traditional yoga philosophy states that the yogi's mind is undisturbed by the opposing forces of pleasure and pain, attachment and aversion. Instead of reacting to the inner or outer world, the yogi maintains a peaceful, equanimous disposition at all times. This is an integral part of the practice. Just as core strength and flexibility are things you practice each time you get on your mat, the true practice of a yoga-applied life is about training your mind to remain balanced amid all the vicissitudes of life.

Upekshanam is the observational quality of mind that inhabits the space between the stimulus and the conditioned response to that stimulus. Equanimity is the freedom to choose enlightened action above action based solely on personal preferences. Contrary to what you might see on social media, yoga practice is often a struggle. You come to your mat and fail numerous times before finally succeeding. Some poses, like deep backbends, are actually designed to provoke heightened emotional responses and to stimulate subconscious triggers. Yoga gives you a structure in which to work through these obstacles. There have been countless times in my life when the practice of asanas has triggered intense emotions for me. I've been caught up in anger, depression, anxiety, panic, and frustration—at times to a debilitating degree. But thankfully, by retraining my mind to remain equanimous, I have gained the strength to live a more peaceful and balanced life.

If you think that your practice should always feel a certain way or that your life should be a certain way, then you will bind yourself into the realm of "should." The body is part of the ever-changing world of impermanence and is beyond this realm. Patanjali's Yoga Sutras offer freedom that is transcendent from *sukha* (pleasure) and *dukha* (pain). We cannot, according to Patanjali, define the success of our practice by the experience of pleasure or pain. We must find transcendent peace from an equanimous mind. Reality simply is what it is. The story we tell around reality and how we react to the various triggers that stimulate our nervous system are chains that tie us to cycles of misery.

Emotions are like storms that obscure the natural clarity of the mind. If you only heed the call of your emotions, you will often find yourself making decisions that lead to physical, mental, or emotional suffering. Patanjali's Yoga Sutras advise yogis to cultivate an equanimous mind in the presence of anyone or anything that we designate as evil or wrong—essentially anything that gets our blood boiling. The yogi's task is to remain centered and to walk the thin line between pleasure and pain. In other words, Patanjali echoes what most contemporary psychotherapists advise: take no action when you're triggered. First, reclaim your composure and prepare to take action only when your mind is clear. This simple, humble teaching can transform your life. Once your mind is calm, you see clearly and can wait for the appropriate action and response to come to you. Equanimity is the ultimate strength because once you have your mind and emotions under control, nothing can ever disturb your spiritual center.

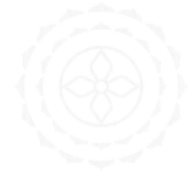

1. Take the anger antidote. When we act out of anger, we only harm ourselves. Yelling at someone in an effort to prove we're right means that even if we win the argument, we still lose because of the residual damage done to ourselves and our relationship. Learn how to disengage whenever you're flooded with emotion and cannot see clearly. Learn how not to take the emotional bait in an argument. If you can't see straight, how can you engage in an enlightened action? Ask yourself where you have been acting out of anger, righteous indignation, or just a feeling that the other person was wrong. See if you can take a step back and cultivate equanimity instead. It takes great strength to drop the fight and walk away. Once you regain your calm mind, ask for guidance about the next step and wait to act until it comes from a place of love. Walking away is not quitting if you make a commitment to return once you regain your composure.

2. Practice equanimity toward yourself. It's easy to judge yourself harshly and to internalize anger and frustration. Watch your inner dialogue, and each time you notice yourself engaging in self-directed negativity, move the tone away from judgment and toward the center line of pure observation. Cultivate equanimous thoughts toward yourself. Observe yourself without any tinge of emotionality. If you're tired, observe that tiredness is present. If you're happy, observe that happiness is present. If you're angry, observe that anger is present. Do not fight or control; just observe with a calm, equanimous mind.

3. Identify your triggers. Which yoga poses press your buttons, and why? Which people in your life annoy you the most, and why? Which life situations are hardest for you to handle, and why? Knowing where you need to work on equanimity helps prepare for the test once it's at hand. As soon as you feel yourself triggered, bring your mind back to a neutral point of observation such as the breath. Take no action until you feel centered again.

PRACTICE

1. *Sukhasana*—Comfortable Seated Pose

Cross your legs and sit on the ground as comfortably as possible. Bring the mind's point of attention to your breath. Cultivate an equanimous mind by remaining free from judgment. Simply observe the experience of the breath with no expectation or attachment for any particular experience. After five minutes, place your hands in prayer position and end by resonating the sound OM.

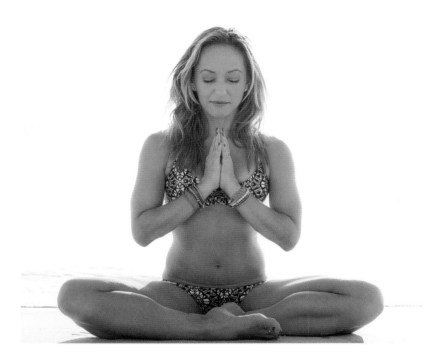

2. *Adho Mukha Vrksasana*—Straight Line Handstand

A straight handstand—the epitome of perfect equilibrium—is actually a balance between strength and flexibility. Remain equanimous while attempting to balance in a handstand. Let go of your attachment to the goal of the shape and simply observe the experience. If you don't have a solid handstand, the best way to start is by performing this pose against a wall to assist with alignment and help build your strength. If you decide to use the wall, get as close as possible to it so you can align the back of your head, your glutes, and maybe even the back of your rib cage.

When you're ready try it without the wall, kick up to a handstand and find the vertical line through your body. Externally rotate your shoulders to push your arms away from your head. Elevate your shoulder blades and press up with your shoulders. It should feel like your shoulders are touching your ears. Draw your lower ribs in, engage your legs, and point your toes. Squeeze your glutes and find the balance point along your center line. Gaze at the ground between your hands. Stay here for at least five breaths.

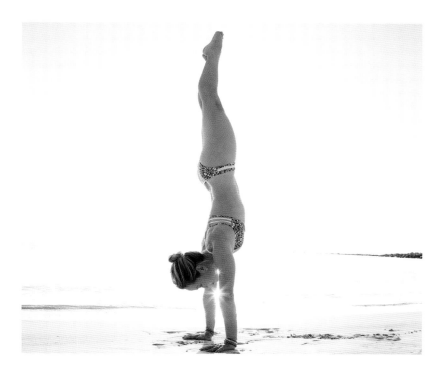

3. *Kapotasana*—Pigeon Pose

Many students find that Kapotasana challenges their inner sense of equanimity. This deep backbend triggers a heightened state of emotional arousal and often brings up anxiety, panic, anger, or sadness. Rather than running away and avoiding these emotions, students are encouraged to cultivate an equanimous mind in the face of adversity. This effort retrains the nervous system and makes the equanimous mind more accessible in life situations that trigger similar emotional responses.

Start in a kneeling position. Inhale to create space as you lift your ribs away from your hips, send your pelvis forward, elevate your sternum, and reach your hands over your head. You may need to stop at this point if you reach a physical or emotional limit. If so, respect that and remain equanimous. Take five breaths and then rest in Balasana (Child's Pose). From a kneeling position fold forward while keeping your knees bent and tucked into your chest. Allow your head to gently touch the floor ahead of the knees and drape your arms by your sides.

When you're ready to attempt the full expression of Kapotasana, exhale as you reach your hands toward your feet, eventually wrapping your fingers fully around your heels or your calves. Place your elbows on the ground in line with your shoulders. Rotate your hips inward and your shoulders outward. Suck in your lower belly. Stay here for five breaths as you gaze at your nose. Inhale as you release your heels and place your hands on the ground next to each foot; stay here for another five breaths. Inhale and return to a kneeling position. Take Balasana if you need to rest, or jump back to Chaturanga Dandasana. Inhale and come forward to Urdhva Mukha Svanasana, then exhale and roll back to Adho Mukha Svanasana.

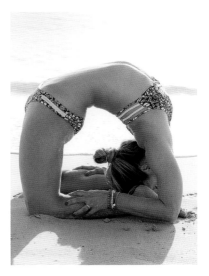
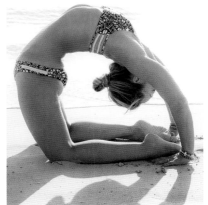

4. *Samanasana*—Balancing Prana Pose

This pose is harder than it looks. The name comes from the root word *samana*—meaning the balancing energy, or *prana*—and this pose seeks to create a strong sense of inner balance and an orientation toward the center line. If you deviate at all from that line, you will roll off to the side. Samanasana is a simple looking yet humbling pose that teaches you the physical state of the center line.

Start off in a supine position; roll over onto your right side. Place your right hand under your body. Keep the side of your right foot on the ground and stack your left foot on top of the right. Press your head into the ground. Inhale as you extend your left arm and balance here. If you are able to maintain the balance, extend your left leg up and wrap your fingers around your left big toe. It is also possible to bend your knee to grab the toe; however, this may disturb the balance. If you cannot reach your toe, you can simply raise your arm. Stabilize your core, point your left toes, and look up at your left foot. Stay here for five breaths. Release and repeat on the other side.

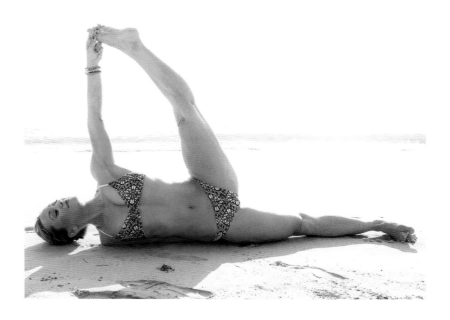

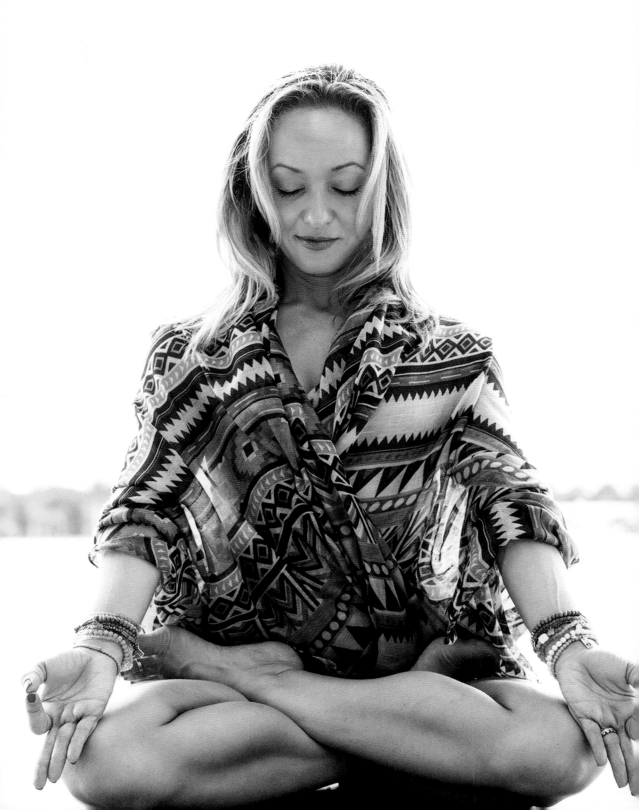

Day 9 | The Magic of the Breath
Prana

The real star of every yoga practice is the breath. You do not need a fancy place to practice or to be a master of handstands (although those are fun!) to drop your mind into a state of powerful presence. All you need is an open heart. Inner peace is never more than a few breaths away. Taking time each day to reconnect with your breath grounds your mind and emotions and anchors your inner awareness. Breath awareness is like an inner barometer for your emotional state. Short, shallow breaths may indicate a heightened state of emotion. A deep sigh may indicate a state of release, sadness, or relaxation. Regular, sustained breath may indicate focus and concentration. As you know your breath, so too will you know your mind, body, and emotions.

Today's yogi assignment is the breath, called *prana* in Sanskrit. More than just oxygen, the breath is associated with the *prana vayu*, the winds of our life force, and focusing on the breath can elicit a deep experience of the true self within. The *vinyasa* method of Ashtanga Yoga is based on the coordination of breath with movement. Shri K. Pattabhi Jois always said that yoga is really a breathing practice. The breath is the key to training the mind. Having an untrained mind is like flipping TV channels—thoughts and emotions are "shows" constantly playing on the inner screen of the mind. Yoga teaches you how to change the channel and find a "program" you like instead of letting the mind run wild. The solution to reining in your mind is deceptively simple—turn your attention to where you want it to go. Carefully train the mind by first focusing on the breath and then turning your attention inward. Steadily focusing on the breath invites the mind to feel the inner body. Just as the body itself can be felt in increasingly more refined layers, so too can the breath be felt in more refined and rarefied forms.

But remaining steadfastly focused on the breath is not an easy task. During asana practice, the yoga poses themselves can be a distraction.

In the midst of life, there is an endless sea of distractions. The first step in maintaining unbroken awareness on the breath is practicing the state of concentration called *dharana* in Sanskrit, the fifth limb of the Ashtanga Yoga method. Dharana consists of efforts aimed at steadying and strengthening the mind. Meditation—*dhyana* in Sanskrit—is the sixth limb of the Ashtanga Yoga method, and it is a thoughtless, wordless state into which you can slip only after the mind is focused on a single point of attention. The ability of the mind to remain focused on a single point of attention is a clear measure of the power of the yogi's mind. This attention is called the *eka tattva* state, also known as the meditative mind or the yogi's mind. Calm, balanced, and equanimous, the yogi's mind is able to remain focused on a single point of attention over a sustained period of time. It is only the calm mind that can experience the deepest truth of the spirit within. Start off with the humble task of being steady and single-pointed for ten deep breaths and then expand the power of the mind.

Sitting for five minutes with unbroken awareness on the breath can be harder for many people than working on yoga poses. However, if you start with this simple task and let it initiate your journey into the yogi's mind, it will transform not only your asana practice but also your whole life. There may be times when you will not be able to perform asanas, but there will never be a time while you are alive when you are not breathing. When I was thirty years old, my father was resuscitated from two heart attacks, had a triple bypass operation, and got a defibrillator installed. After the second heart attack, he woke up to find himself intubated, without any memory of the heart attack or procedure, and unable to move. Earlier that year, he had joined a meditation course in which I taught the technique of focusing on the breath to steady the mind in moments of great distress. After he could speak again, my father told me the only thing that kept his mind calm and free from panic was to think of the simple tool of bringing his attention to his breath. He kept his mind on the simple awareness of inhalation and exhalation and away from the chaos happening in his own body.

My husband, Tim Feldmann, taught yoga to combat war veterans who suffered from post-traumatic stress disorder (PTSD). One of these brave soldiers took to the yoga breathing technique above everything else. After his first experience with deep breathing, he told Tim that he felt "like before the war." He said that his nervous system was so jacked up from the wartime stress that he had forgotten what it felt like to be "normal." After he had been practicing for a few months, he shared with Tim that during a PTSD attack at home, when ordinarily he would have been stuck for hours until his wife came home, he applied the deep breathing technique he had learned in yoga class and was able to regain his balance and calm.

There are countless stories about the transformative power of the breath, and I invite you to experience that power for yourself. Let ten deep breaths be an invitation to your inner world and a place of peace within yourself. An untrained mind will often veer toward negativity—fear, drama, anger, unhappiness, desire, dissatisfaction, a general sense of malaise, irritability, self-pity, and self-loathing. These are the resting points of the untrained mind and the root of suffering. By focusing on the breath, you are willing to surrender to something bigger and let the old ways go. Focusing on the breath gives you a tool that you can pull out in times of need, like when you're stressed, tired, upset, or just generally annoyed. The ability to take ten deep breaths can change your life. With a strong, steady mind, keep your attention on the path and take one small step forward every day. With devotion, discipline, and determination, there is nothing you can't accomplish.

HOMEWORK

1. Practice breath awareness. At some point today, pause and take stock of your current state. Then close your eyes, sit still, and consciously follow the breath for a slow, steady count of ten. Count your breaths backward, saying, "Ten in, nine in, eight in," all the way down to one as you inhale; do the same type of count as you exhale. Start or end your asana practice with this breath awareness, or take a few minutes for it while you're at work or right before you get home. You can also take some mental space at the end of the day or before responding to an important communication. After just ten conscious breaths, open your eyes and take stock of your current situation again.

2. Take a stress antidote. The next time you feel overwhelmed with stress, press pause on the console of your mind and take ten deep breaths. Instead of arguing or reacting as you normally would in sticky situations, train yourself to always take ten deep, conscious breaths before acting. Think about how many personal wars could have been avoided and how much more love and light there would be in the world if people didn't immediately surrender to their emotional, in-the-moment reactions. Wait for the next time you are triggered and then be strong enough to walk away and take ten deep breaths.

3. The breath body—Through deep breathing techniques based on Ujjayi Pranayama in Ashtanga Yoga, you gain access to the natural state of a calm, clear, and present mind. Start to apply this deep breathing to your asana practice. It is the deceptively simple movement that holds the key to yoga's magic. Sometimes called the Darth Vader Breath, the Ocean Breath, or the Victorious Breath, the deep breathing with sound that defines the Ashtanga Yoga method offers you a tool that can transform your life.

Sit in a comfortable position with your spine straight. Engage your pelvic floor and draw your subnavel into your body. Seal your lips, close the epiglottis a little, and elongate the breath to a maximum of ten seconds on the inhalation and ten seconds on the exhalation. Let the sound SA resonate with the inhalation and the sound HA with the exhalation. Match the length of inhalation with that of the exhalation. Breathe ten times. By opening a channel into the subtle awareness of the inner body, ten deep breaths can reset your nervous system and return you to a state of calm.

PRACTICE

1. *Padmasana*—Lotus Pose

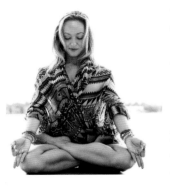

Finding a basic, comfortable seated position is harder than it sounds at first. Most people spend the majority of their time sitting on chairs and sofas and not so much sitting on the ground. Spending at least five minutes a day in a seated position will gently encourage your hips to open, strengthen your spine, and facilitate breathing from the diaphragm.

Sit in a simple cross-legged position, or if your hips are already open, sit in Padmasana. Remain still, without moving, for around five minutes. Draw the mind's point of attention to your breath. Refine the area of your attention to the space inside your nostrils, along your upper lip, and around your nose. If you notice thoughts coming and going, just ask the mind to come back. If you feel strong emotions that draw your attention, just ask the mind to come back. If you feel intense physical sensations, do your best to maintain the same position and refrain from moving. Remain calm and equanimous, and keep your mind free of any value judgments of the breath. Once you bring your attention to your breath, employ the deep yoga breathing technique explained earlier for ten conscious breaths.

2. Constructive Rest Pose

Start in a supine position. Bend your knees and place your feet about hip-width apart. Allow your knees to fold in toward each other. Place your sacrum flat on the ground and draw your shoulder blades under your upper back. Drape your hands either on your lower belly or comfortably by your hips. Close your eyes. Breathe deeply, in and out through your nose, allowing your belly

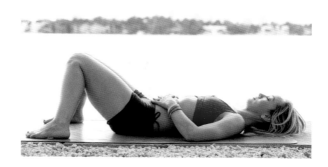

to rise and flatten with each cycle of the breath. Count backward from ten in coordination with the breath. Say the words "Ten in" and "Ten out" to keep the mind steady. (Note that this breathing technique is used solely for relaxation and is not applicable during physical asana practice.) Repeat as many times as you like. Practice this technique whenever you feel stressed or have lower back pain.

3. *Savasana*—Corpse Pose

In the Ashtanga tradition this pose is often known simply as "take rest." Savasana is the pose of final relaxation in which your mind is focused inward and your body restores itself. Lie down on your back. Spread your feet a little more than hip-width apart. Allow your legs to flop open in a natural external rotation. Place your sacrum flat on the ground, and draw your shoulder blades under your upper back. Allow your arms to lie out to the sides and turn your palms up. Close your eyes. Focus on your breath. Do not try to control or manipulate the breath in any way. Keep your attention confined to the subtle sensations of the inner body. Remain here for between five and twenty minutes. Hold this pose at the end of every yoga practice and whenever you feel in need of rest throughout the day.

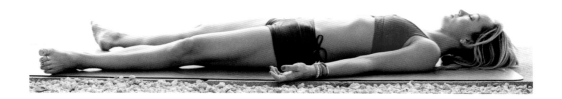

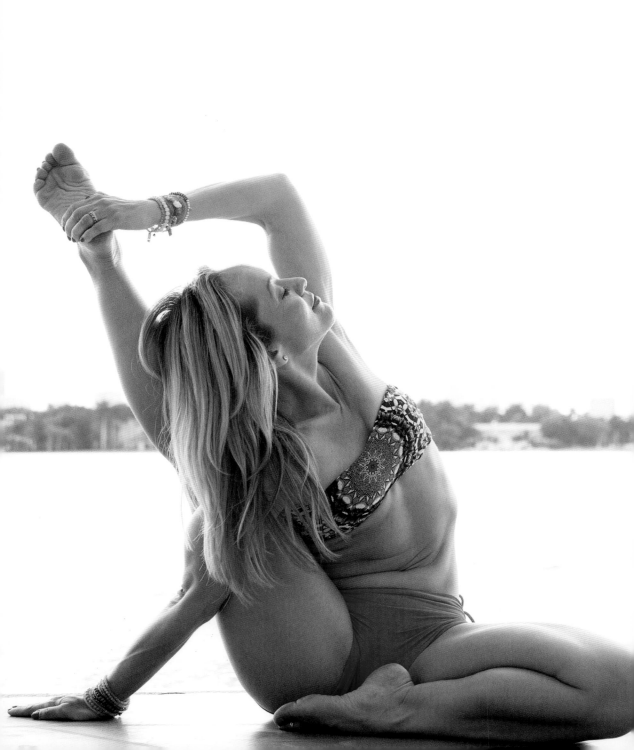

Day 10 | Truthfulness and Authenticity
Satya

Today's yogi assignment is authenticity. The Sanskrit word *satya*, usually translated as "truthfulness," can also mean "authenticity." When you wake up one day and realize that all you need to be is yourself, then you are finally free. If you spend your life being what you think you should be or what other people want you to be, then you will always feel empty on some level. There is something so captivating about people who unapologetically own their truth. You are a divine creation—blessed, whole, and complete. You do not need to be the first, the biggest, the loudest, or the best. You just need to be yourself!

In my life, I have struggled to remain strong, authentic, and coura-geously myself—especially since entering the public sphere as a teacher. It can be very scary to be yourself in public, with countless people watch-ing your every move. By putting yourself out there, you risk negative feedback from anonymous strangers, and it is too easy to start taking that in and doubting yourself. Staying true to yourself and being authentic is the only sane way to live. In my yoga career, I've been called many things, including vapid, hollow, fake, fame-seeking, privileged, ignorant, uninformed, uneducated, and intimidating. Add to that a whole series of comments about my butt, feet, cellulite, and age, and it could be a recipe for a self-esteem disaster. Men send me inappropriate images and leave illicit comments about me on social media. I've even thought about retreating and taking down all my social media accounts, but I realize that is not the solution. In my life and in yours, the solution is to live as genuinely, "heartfully," and courageously as possible. Love what you do each day, and stay true to yourself. Be fierce and fearless.

Close your eyes, take a deep breath, and say these words out loud to yourself: "I am worthy. I am enough. I am filled with unconditional love." Say them again. It is the truth. Do not let anyone tell you otherwise. There is nothing you need to do to be worthy of love. There is nothing you can do to revoke your spiritual inheritance. You are worthy. You are enough. You are filled with unconditional love. You just need to open your eyes, soften your heart, and let it all in. Give yourself permission to be exactly who you are. Relax, let go, and just be yourself.

HOMEWORK

1. Stop people-pleasing. Think about how many times in your life you have modified your behavior or edited yourself to please someone else or to try to prove that you're a good person. Take a moment and validate yourself. You *are* a good person. You're doing the best you can. You're not perfect, but your heart is in the right place. Be yourself. Be true to yourself. Be strong enough to take the good and the bad and not let it take you off your authentic course. Don't change to please people. Sing the tune of you, with the relaxed self-acceptance that comes from knowing exactly who you are.

2. Haters gonna hate; don't negotiate. Identify mean-spirited people and comments, and do not engage with them. Do not try to win anyone over to the light. Don't waste your time thinking about nasty comments meant only to disparage and hurt you. Set clear boundaries and do not engage with the haters. Do not respond to nasty comments on social media; delete ranting emails with no purpose other than to draw you in; break all ties and do not take the emotional bait. But if someone offers you constructive criticism aimed at making you a better person, reflect on it and do not defend yourself. But do not automatically change to please anyone. Be strong enough to be authentically yourself.

3. Don't be sorry. There is no right way to be yourself. Just be yourself and don't apologize for it. Don't waste another breath excusing your-self for your greatness because it makes someone else feel small. That's not to say that if you've done something wrong, you shouldn't offer a sincere apology—you should. But stop apologizing for being yourself.

1. *Utthita Parsvakonasana A*—Extended Side-Angle Pose

Simple standing poses such as Utthita Parsvakonasana A form the basis of the yoga practice. Spending time feeling rooted through your legs and working on cultivating an inner sense of spaciousness through your pelvic floor gives you a firm basis in your center. The gentle external rotation of the hips activated in Utthita Parsvakonasana A is both approachable and challenging.

Inhale as you step your feet one leg-length apart. This distance is adjustable based on your height, leg length, and level of flexibility. Turn your left foot out so the left heel aligns with your right arch. Exhale as you bend your left knee over your left ankle, moving toward the middle of your foot. Be sure your knee does not reach beyond your toes. Slide your torso down toward your left thigh, and lay your upper body along the outer edge of the thigh as your left hand reaches toward the ground. Align your left hand with the outer edge of your left foot; root either your fingertips or your whole hand into the ground. Press firmly back into your right foot. Inhale as you extend your right arm over your head, following the line of the right side of your body to fully enter Utthita Parsvakonasana A. Draw in your lower ribs, suck your belly back into the inner space of your pelvis, firm your right leg, straighten your arms, and gaze toward your right fingers. Avoid dipping your hips too low; instead, keep the left thigh parallel to the ground at a maximum. Stay in the pose for five breaths, then repeat on the right side.

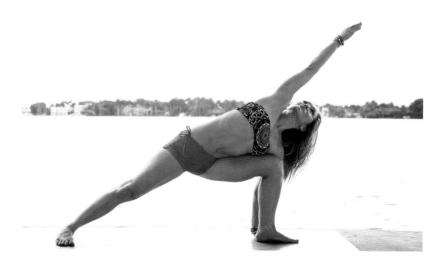

2. *Marichyasana A—Pose Dedicated to Sage Marichi A*

Named after the great sage Marichi, this seated pose is a powerful hip and lower back opener, which also allows you to drop your attention deeply inward. Finding the inner body is a key step in knowing who you are. Poses like Marichyasana A help you maintain your spiritual center.

Start in Dandasana. Inhale as you bend your right knee and place your foot flat on the ground with the knee pointing straight up. Align your right heel with the outer edge of your right hip, and keep a hand width between your right foot and your left thigh. Exhale as you reach your torso forward, aligning your sternum with your left knee. Rotate your right shoulder inward as you wrap your right arm around your right shinbone. Bend your right elbow around your right thigh. Reach your left arm up and bend the elbow back without rotating your shoulders outward. Interlace your fingers behind your back, or grab one wrist with the other hand. If you cannot bind your hands together, use a towel or strap to complete the pose. Ground the right side of your hips, but do not force the right sitting bone down to the floor. Fold your chin toward your left shin and gaze toward your toes. Stay here for five breaths. Release and repeat on the left side.

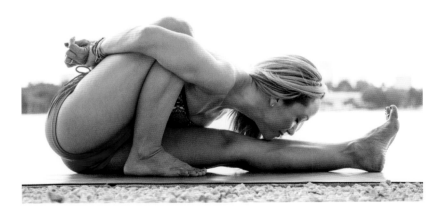

3. *Parivrtta Surya Yantrasana—Compass Pose*

Parivrtta Surya Yantrasana is a powerful hip, hamstring, and lower back opener that demands that you find your inner sense of direction. Much like a compass always tells you where true north lies, the inner compass always tells you where your authentic sense of self lies. Parivrtta Surya Yantrasana is a very challenging pose that requires a high level of flexibility, so do not be impatient or rush the journey. Instead, be truthful with your limits and practice accepting them.

Start off in a simple seated pose with your legs crossed. Inhale as you lift your right leg off the ground and slide your right shoulder forward in front of your right knee. Bend your right knee around your right shoulder. Hold on to your right calf muscle with your right hand, and reach your left hand over your head to hold your right heel. Settle your sitting bones on the ground and avoid hiking up your right hip for added leverage. Exhale as you place your right hand on the ground out to the side for support and straighten the elbow. Inhale as you suck in your lower belly and create space deep within your pelvic floor to allow your right thighbone to drop deeper into its socket. Exhale as you straighten your right leg, pull firmly with your left arm, ground your sitting bones, and twist your torso. If you cannot straighten your leg yet, simply hold your right foot and straighten your leg as much as possible. Allow the right side of your rib cage to drop in while the left side goes up. Look up toward your right foot. Stay here for five breaths. Release and repeat on the left side.

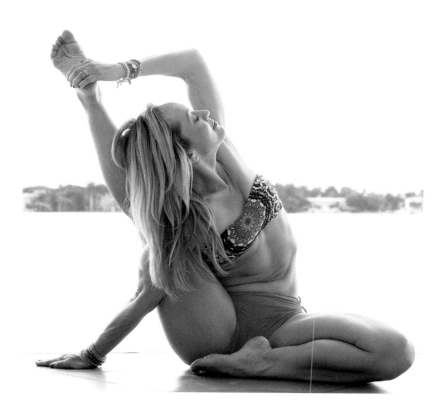

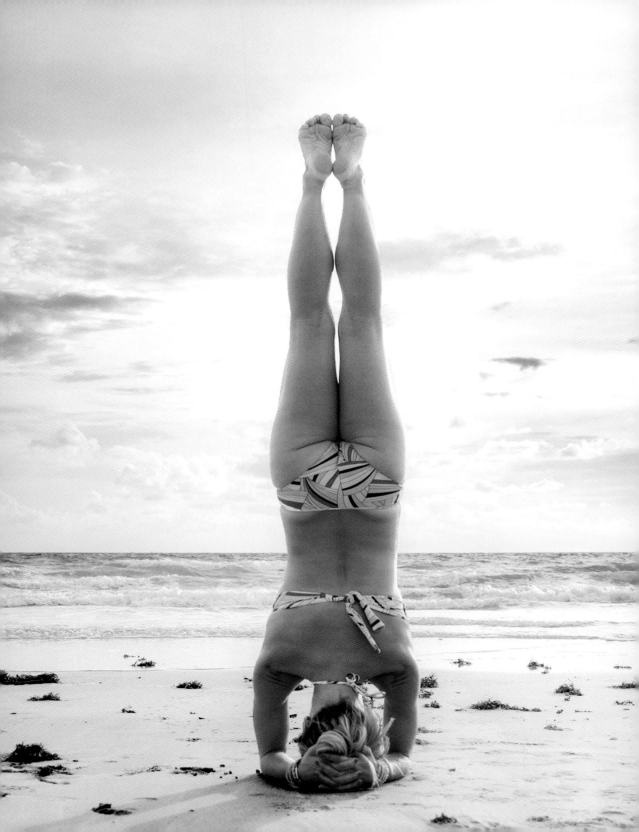

Intention
Sankalpa

I woke up one day seventeen years ago with a sincere desire to live a more peaceful life. Late nights and nameless substitutes for intimacy led me to an emotional dead end. I was young and haughty, full of pride and false invincibility. I left a trail of misery and drama behind me without realizing the repercussions of my selfish actions. I lived in a spiritual black hole. My first step down the path of yoga came out of a yearning to change my world and to bring love and trust back to my barren emotional landscape.

Today's yogi assignment is intention, or *sankalpa*. Once my intention was set toward the yoga life, my world slowly started to change, one breath at a time. I went to India; traded parties for practice; and shifted selfishness to generosity, cynicism to understanding, and depression to love. You can do it too. You just need to set your intention with your full heart.

Setting a clear intention helps prevent you from veering off course in life. Everyone has an inherent moral compass that values certain things above others. We rarely get our most effective motivation from material pleasures. Instead, our most profound and powerful dreams are about hope, peace, and love. Setting your intention along the deeper meaning of every path you follow is one small thing you can do to create the right conditions for a happy and peaceful life. When my husband and I wanted to open a yoga center in Miami, we knew that our intention wasn't to get rich. We wanted to create a home for the authentic, traditional practice of Ashtanga Yoga. There were many temptations that might have earned us money more quickly, but we were clear about our intention. A clear intention is the benchmark against which you can measure all your decisions. If something does not align with your intention, then you simply do not act on it. The most successful people I have met in life are those with the clearest intentions and the integrity to stay true to their core values.

The first step in living the life you want is to recognize and acknowledge your biggest and boldest dream. Do not worry right now how it's going to come true or think about all the obstacles in your way. Don't overthink it—just dream with your heart. If your dream scares you with its potential of success, then you know it's the one you have to embrace! You don't need to share your dream with anyone yet (unless you want to), and it doesn't matter if someone else is already doing what you want to do. Your dream is yours, and the simple act of owning it (even if it's only privately) generates a whole wave of energy that will set you in motion. You will be drawn forward down the path of intention.

HOMEWORK

1. Write it down. Dream your wildest dream. Ask yourself this question: What would you do if you knew there was no possibility of failure? Write it down on a piece of paper or in a Word document, date it, and save it. Don't worry about the pragmatics or the logistics. Just dream.

2. Examine your yogi heart. Ask yourself what your intention is with your practice. Why do you practice yoga? Or if you don't yet practice, ask yourself what inspires you about the yoga life. Dig deep within yourself to find your heart's intention for living the yogi's life.

3. Find your core values. Identifying your personal core values will set the deeper intention for your life. Make a list of the qualities that have profound personal meaning for you. Do not follow anyone else's idea of what has meaning. Be truly honest with yourself about what you value. For example, after many years of introspection, I realized that beauty is something that has intrinsic value for me, so I honor it in my life. I like beautiful things and enjoy making myself look beautiful. Beauty for me is material, spiritual, energetic, and emotional. It is the experience of life at its best, a perfect sunrise after a dark night, a rainbow after a torrential downpour, generosity amid suffering, and strength through adversity. Beauty is the awe-inspiring harmony of Beethoven's symphonies, the taste of a ripe mango, the feeling you get when someone smiles at you. Some people might consider me superficial to value beauty, but to me, it is an expression of the magic of life.

1. *Baddha Hasta Sirsasana A*—Bound Hand Headstand

Standing on my head isn't something I ever thought I would do on a regular basis. In fact, when I started yoga practice, I was so bad at headstands that I had to try repeatedly for almost a year before I could balance. There were many days when I felt defeated, but slowly I developed a small kernel of faith. That little seed eventually grew into strength. The journey of strength is about setting your intention, putting in the work every day, and never giving up.

Start off on your hands and knees. Place your elbows on the ground hip-width apart and interlock your fingers, keeping your palms open. Stabilize your shoulder girdle. Exhale as you place the top of your head on the ground between your palms. Straighten your legs up and walk your feet in as close to your head as possible. Thrust into your elbows, draw in your lower ribs, and engage your pelvic floor. Inhale as you send your hips forward over the foundation of your arms and allow your legs to lift. When your legs are parallel to the ground, tuck your tailbone, firm your quadriceps, and align your body along the vertical axis to fully enter Baddha Hasta Sirsasana A. Stay here for ten to twenty breaths, then come down. Rest in Balasana. If you cannot balance in a headstand, hold the preparation for the entire count with your hips stacked over shoulders and your feet still on the ground. Do not use the wall; just hold the pose until you are strong enough to come up into the pose.

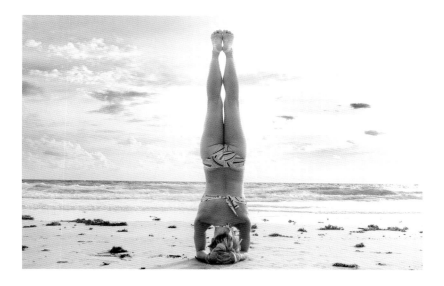

2. *Mukta Hasta Sirsasana C*—Unsupported Headstand

This is one of the most challenging headstands in the Ashtanga Yoga practice. It requires a strong mind, firm shoulders, and a well-aligned core to find your balance here. Set your intention to orient toward the center line, and you will slowly make your way into Mukta Hasta Sirsasana C.

Start in Adho Mukha Svanasana. Exhale as you place the top of your head on the ground by bending your arms and slowly lowering down. Keep your knees off the ground, but if necessary, you can set them down long enough to find the center line. With your head on the ground, slowly move your arms out to the side, palms down. Ideally your hands should align with your shoulders, but you may find it easier to balance if you place your hands just slightly in front of your shoulders. Inhale as you lift your hips and walk your feet forward. Send your hips forward, grip your fingertips into the ground, and pivot through your hip joints to lift to the vertical line. Stay here for five breaths. Switch your hands to the tripod stance and exhale as you jump all the way back to Chaturanga Dandasana. If you cannot balance in headstand, hold the preparation with your hips stacked over shoulders and your feet on the ground for the entire count.

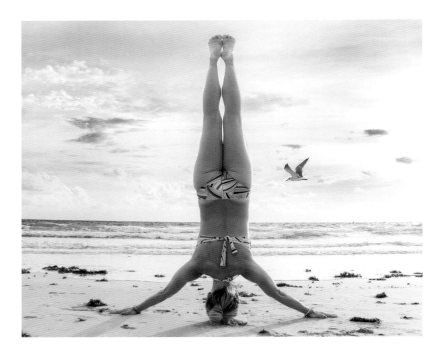

3. *Utpluthih*—Sprung Up

The literal translation of *Utpluthih* is "sprung up," and you will need a strong intention, willpower, and determination to succeed in this pose. You may also see this pose called Tolasana in Sanskrit, which means Scales Pose. Shri K. Pattabhi Jois used to ask his students to hold this pose while he counted to ten. But he never counted in numerical order. He always skipped numbers and repeated sequences, sometimes going from nine all the way back to five. It often broke my determination to listen to his meandering count. Then one day I set my intention to stay for the full ten count, no matter what. The first thing I had to do was stop paying attention to the count and focus on my inner work. By clearly stating my intention, I got the strength and discipline to hold what was often nearly one hundred breaths in this challenging pose. By setting a strong intention, you will find what it takes to stay for the full count in Utpluthih and stay with your intentions in everyday life.

Start by folding your legs into Padmasana or simply cross your legs. Take your hands slightly in front of your hips and align them on the ground at about midthigh. Exhale as you stabilize your shoulder girdle and engage your pelvic floor.

Inhale as you engage your lower abdominal muscles and lift your hips. Press firmly with your arms, bring your hips up toward your ribs, and shorten your torso. Draw your lower ribs in and fold into the center line. Keep your head in a neutral position, gaze at your nose, and use your abdominal muscles to lift up into Utpluthih. Stay here for at least ten deep breaths. Set your intention, and do not give up. If you cannot immediately lift up, just keep pushing into the ground using the technique outlined here, and one day you will!

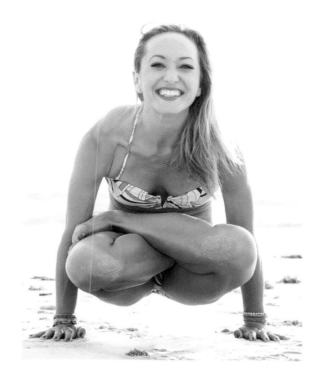

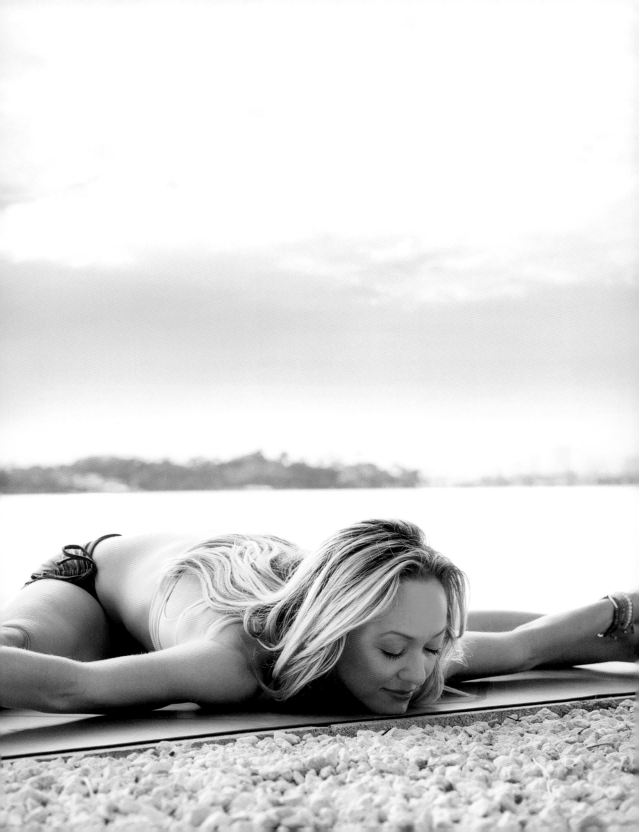

Directing the Senses
Pratyahara

Today's yogi assignment is *pratyahara*, which is traditionally understood as "sense withdrawal" or "sense control." What does it mean to have control over your senses, and why is this important in yoga practice?

Cultivating pratyahara is the fifth limb along the eight-limbed path of Ashtanga Yoga. Yoga philosophy portrays the five traditional senses as five horses that draw the chariot of the body. The mind is considered to be the chariot driver. But just as a charioteer must have command over the horses so they will not go rogue, the yogi must retain control over the organs of the five senses so they will not usurp the role of the driver. An epic struggle between the material and the spiritual worlds takes place through the organs of the five senses; the yogi's task is to attain mastery over the senses and keep control in life. When you have little control of your responses to external stimuli, it leads to an action/reaction cycle that is tied to the material world. With no space between stimulus and response, you are essentially defined by the nature of your experience. So you will naturally run after pleasure and run away from pain.

While it may be tempting to think you can just turn off your senses, much like you would switch off a television, the yogic training of pratyahara is achieved through a conscious redirection of the faculties of the senses to the inner body. When this happens, the senses appear to stop or withdraw from the external world. Far more than a mere on-off switch of the sense organs, pratyahara retrains those organs to focus on the subtle world that lies just under the surface layer of awareness. It is actually the knowledge gleaned from this shift in perspective that is the deeper goal of pratyahara. When the sense organs remain singularly attentive to the inner experience, a wealth of knowledge arises. Imagine you were able to perceive the smallest, most infinitesimal atom in your body and actually "see" it. The yogi's mind has that power through inner sight. Inner sight brings the brilliant imagery of the body and the subconscious mind to conscious awareness.

Similarly, inner feeling—kinesthetic sensitivity along the deepest layers of the body—opens a path to a world of sensations that often elude description, such as the ineffable feeling of lightness, emptiness, and resplendence as though whole universes are contained within the body. Inner hearing allows you to tune in to the quiet voice of wisdom that yearns to speak to you from your heart center. Inner taste and smell are perhaps harder to train but operate in the same capacity. It could be said that metaphor is the language of the body, and through the cultivation of pratyahara, you develop the power to directly perceive your body's most magical and mystical truths. At its best, pratyahara is like learning a new language that allows you to communicate with your body on its own terms. Unlike intellect, which operates along the clear lines of logic and order, the body is a maze of feeling, wonder, and discovery.

Patanjali states in Yoga Sutra 1.35 that subtle sense perception creates steadiness of mind. Shri K. Pattabhi Jois and R. Sharath Jois encourage students to direct the mind within during practice. They say that pratyahara is complete only when the mind sees God everywhere, feels God everywhere, and experiences God everywhere. But the perception of God is not meant to be an intellectual knowledge; it is meant to be a direct perception of the deepest spiritual truth in the terrain of the subtle body. Following Guruji and Sharath's notion, another way of understanding pratyahara is to break ties with the material world and experience the spiritual world within.

There is a timeless wisdom contained within you. Yoga is an awakening to the truth of who you really are. Once you touch that divine spark within yourself, your world changes. Drop your mind deeper, orient your point of awareness to the seat of the sacred within yourself, and experience a transcendent peace.

1. Enter the subtle body. Sit for five minutes without moving. Close your eyes and feel the subtle vibration just under the surface of your skin. Drop your mind deeper, beyond muscles and tissues into the space between the cells of your body. Start at the top of your head and scan through the inner body with careful attention to detail. Feel your way into the inner world. After passing through your whole body, rest your mind at the center of your sternum. Drop your attention just behind your sternum in the inner body and discover the spiritual heart center. You may feel your physical heart beating or the presence of emotions or an infinite depth that speaks to you out of its profound stillness. Stay for ten breaths in a quiet space of inner listening.

2. Control your senses. Each time the mind gets attracted to something in the external world through a sense organ, consciously redirect your mind to the subtle body. If you hear something that draws your attention, focus on inner hearing. If you see something that draws your attention, focus on inner sight. Contemplate the faculties of the senses so your understanding moves beyond the object of awareness into the field of awareness itself. For example, instead of just hearing what you hear, contemplate the nature of hearing itself.

3. Walk through the inner world. During your next yoga practice, instead of focusing on the overall movements, find one small area of attention in the inner body and direct your mind exclusively there. For example, you might choose to focus your mind on the activation of your pelvic floor and the feeling of emptiness in the center of your pelvic bowl throughout your practice as a root for your field of experience. As your awareness of your pelvic floor deepens, you may find yourself privy to a nearly intangible inner experience.

PRACTICE

1. *Prasarita Padottanasana A*—Wide-Legged Forward Bend
This wide-legged forward fold turns your mind inward and encourages an orientation toward the subtle body.

Start in Samasthiti. Inhale as you step your feet approximately one leg-length apart. This distance is adjustable based on your height, leg length, and level of flexibility. Take your hands to your waist and exhale. Inhale again to create space behind your pubic bone. Exhale as you fold forward. Place your hands on the ground, shoulder-width apart, and align your fingers and toes with each other. Inhale again to create even more space within your pelvic floor. Exhale as you place the top of your head on the ground between your hands. Draw your elbows in to stack them over your wrists. Gaze toward your nose and turn the mind inward. If you cannot get the top of your head to the floor, then simply allow it to point toward the floor. Stay here for five breaths, then inhale and look up. Exhale and firm your pelvic floor. Inhale as you come up, taking your hands to your waist on the way up. Return to Samasthiti.

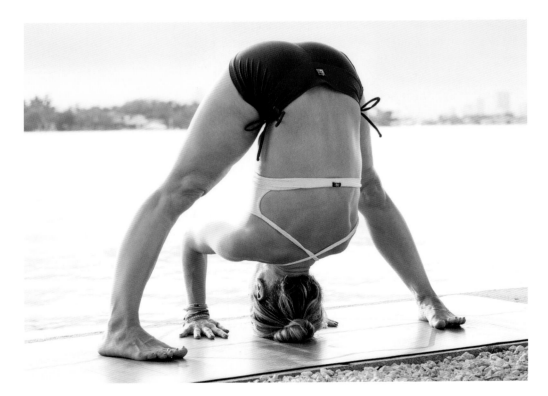

2. *Upavistha Konasana*—Wide-Angle Seated Forward Bend

Keeping your attention rooted in the inner body is crucial for progressing in Upavistha Konasana. Many students start off forcing or pushing themselves to go deeper and thereby expose themselves to hamstring injuries. However, if you draw the mind into an inner state of perception, you will not only practice safely but actually begin to heal your body through your practice.

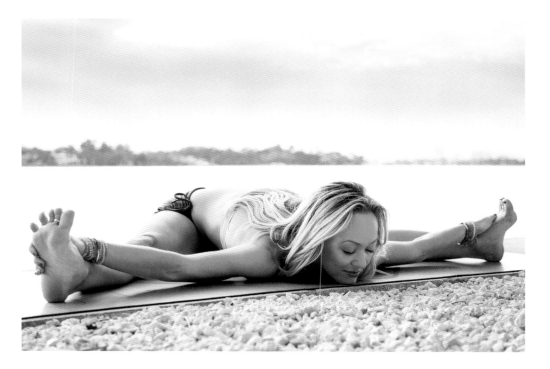

Start off in a seated position, with your legs straight out in front. Inhale as you open your legs in a gentle external rotation to make a V shape. Place your hands on the outer edges of your feet. Spread your feet apart only as far as necessary for your arms to be straight. Keep a sense of spaciousness and hollowness in your pelvic floor to support your hamstrings and lower back. Exhale as you fold your torso down between your thighs. Do *not* pull with your arms. First reach your head toward the ground, then your nose, then your chin, and finally your shoulders and chest.

Do not rush. Gaze at your nose. Stay here for five breaths. If you cannot comfortably hold the outside of your feet, simply rest your hands between your legs and do not attempt to fold forward too deeply. Find a comfortable edge to work and stay there. Inhale as you settle your body weight into the space between your sitting bones and your tailbone. Lift your legs and drop the heads of your thighbones into their sockets. Stretch your legs as far apart as the breadth of your shoulder girdle permits. Look up. Stay here for fives breaths, and then gently come out.

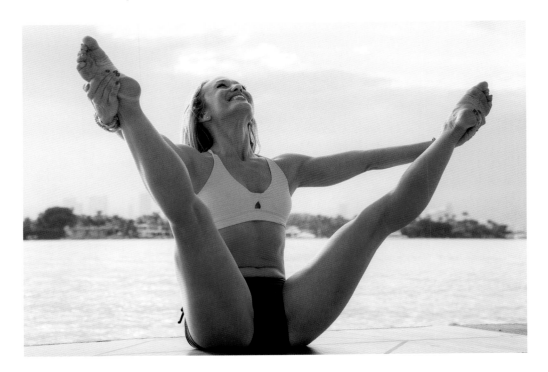

3. *Tittibhasana*—Firefly Pose

The deep hip flexion needed to fold the thighs around the torso demands a drop into the inner state of awareness. Many strong students find Tittibhasana a very challenging pose because you must access this arm balance through the inner body. If you hit it too hard, your legs will simply not get into the right position. Tittibhasana is about attaining the balance and alignment of the magical glow of the firefly itself. Holding this pose for five breaths is a challenging endurance test that brings the mind even deeper within.

Start off in a squatting position. Walk your feet forward outside your arms and step on your hands. Place your calf muscles on top of your upper arms as close to the shoulders as possible and fold your torso forward between your thighs. Sink deep into hip flexion. Press your hands into the ground, and engage your pelvic floor and lower abdominal muscles. Inhale as you firm your shoulder girdle, straighten your arms, and lift your hips off the ground. Straighten your legs while maintaining the lift to fully enter Tittibhasana. If you cannot straighten your legs all the way, then simply straighten them as much as possible. Work with the same technique and keep drawing the heads of your thighbones back into their sockets to ground your legs. Actively draw your thighs toward each other and hug them close to your torso. Keep your lower abdominal muscles firm, and gaze at your nose. Stay here for five breaths, then gently bend your knees and come back down.

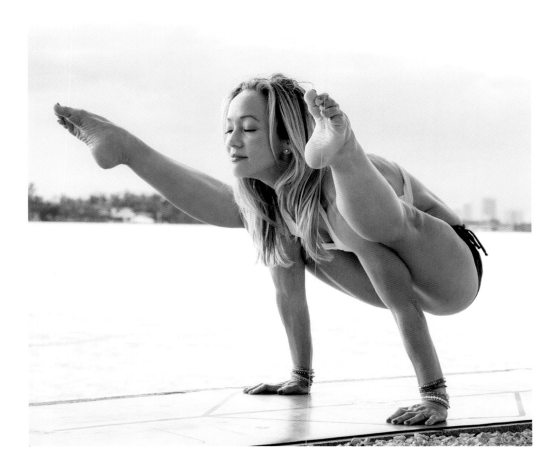

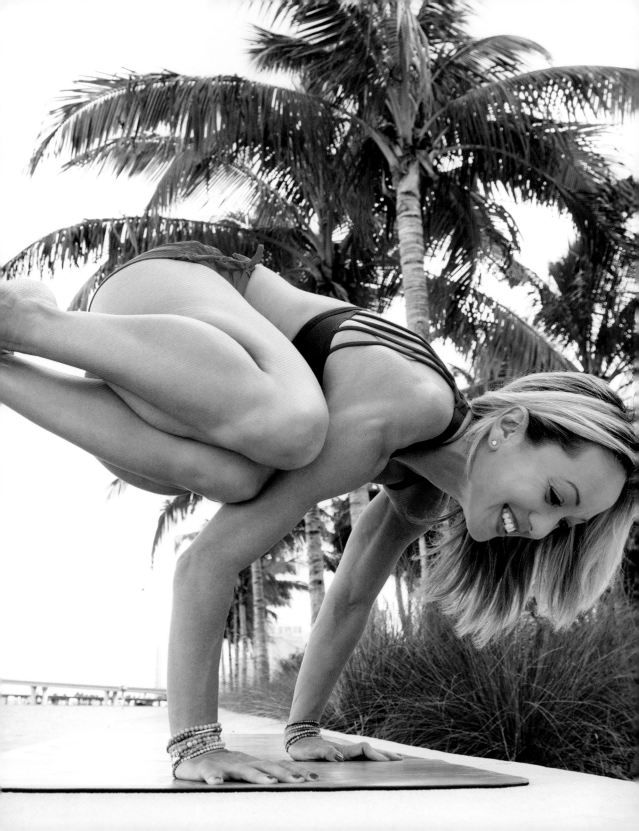

Unshakable Faith
Shraddha

oday's yogi assignment is faith, or *shraddha*. Faith is more than a constructed belief taken on like a rule. In yoga, it is a paradigm, a whole view of the world that, once experienced, changes everything. Built on the highest type of knowledge and born from direct experience, true faith comes with the strength and enthusiasm to work tirelessly for your dreams every single day of your life.

No one is free from the inevitable pains of life, and while it might be tempting to lock down in the face of hardship and fight back against hurt, yoga leads you down a different path. It asks you to trust that everything is going to be okay and that you are strong enough to handle whatever comes your way. Trust begins with recognizing your own basic goodness, a goodness that exceeds the stumbles and falls.

Traditionally, shraddha is presented as the spiritual antidote to doubt. Doubt usually takes one of three forms: you can doubt yourself, your teacher, or the method. You may, for example, find yourself saying that the method is good and the teacher is qualified, but you wonder whether you are really cut out for the practice. Or you may find your-self feeling confident in yourself and the method but questioning your teacher. Or you even may feel that your teacher is qualified and you are proficient, but the method is faulty. Faith is a practice in yoga. First the student demonstrates faith in the method and the teacher. Students make a conscious choice to surrender their personal pref-erences in favor of following a traditional practice. Then, over many years, they cultivate the kernel of faith in themselves. One of the biggest gifts of the practice for me has been the steady cultivation of faith.

Faith also stands in direct opposition to fear. Every breath and every action in life is really rooted in either faith or fear. Acting out of faith produces peace and happiness, whereas acting out of fear results in suffering and pain. Faithful effort leads the yoga practitioner down a balanced road where actions spring forth from a place of deep resolution. Fearful action stems from a feeling of unworthiness that sabotages even the most valiant work. Cultivating faith sometimes means first identifying places where you may be acting out of fear of what you are lacking or from a paradigm in which you chronically doubt yourself.

I never really liked my body. Ever since I can remember, I have been self-conscious about my legs in particular. In middle school, I recall another student calling me "thunder thighs." As a teenager, I would hold my thighs together in the back dreaming of what it would be like to have long, slender thighs instead of my thick ones. I didn't see any of my beauty; all I could see were fat thighs. When I first started yoga, I nearly drowned in a sea of doubt and insecurity. Most of my doubt was self-directed, and most of my effort was based in fear.

At first, yoga seemed to play right into my body-shaming habits. I remember watching in awe as slender yoga goddesses lifted themselves off the ground, while I looked in the mirror and felt wholly inadequate. The more I compared myself to others, the harder I practiced, but the harder I practiced, the more elusive the results seemed to be. Someone described my legs as elephant-sized and suggested that they were just too big to ever lift off the ground. Another student said I could only do deep backbends because my thighs were like big tree trunks. When a very slender colleague suggested that if I were an animal, I would be a frog with thick thighs, I wasn't too thrilled about the reference. All these animalized metaphors fueled my practice from the paradigm of fear. I wondered if what people said was true. Were my thighs really too big to lift? When I did try to raise them, I always carried the seed of doubt and fear with me, and it literally weighed me down. But I never gave up.

I was enamored with the magical appearance of flying in many of the challenging arm balances, handstands, and lift-ups of the yoga practice. And after many years of practice, I remember someone once gave me a compliment that changed how I thought about my body: "Since you have a round body, unlike those lithe yoga goddesses, you've given me hope that I could also lift up." Hearing that statement was a big step in my journey toward accepting my body for what it is, because I realized that I wasn't the only one who felt the way I did. And I also realized that I was strong!

When you can love and accept your whole self, you can love and accept the world. I'm not perfect by any means, but I know that whatever peace I have attained has come to me as the result of daily spiritual practice. Love the shape you are, accept it totally with the knowledge that who you are is perfect and worthy. Take a good, long look at your body insecurities, and cultivate an attitude of acceptance and love. Forgive yourself for all your imperfections, and give yourself permission to be authentically, unapologetically yourself. When I thought I had to look like someone else, act like someone else, and generally conform to some standard of beauty and life that just wasn't me, I felt very inadequate. This led to self-sabotaging behaviors and the basic thought that I wasn't worthy of being loved just as I am. What I really needed was a seed of faith the size of a mustard seed and two magic words: I believe.

So many students have asked me how to overcome doubt. The answer is faith—the kind of faith that says, "I know this to be true because I will work tirelessly to make it so"; the kind of self-knowledge that fills you with the direct experience of the incontrovertible truth of the power and grandness of the universe. The moment you stop worrying about what you look like and start feeling the immeasurable worth of the spirit within you, faith wins over doubt. Now, nearly twenty years older than I was when I first joined a yoga class, I feel more comfortable in my own skin, more beautiful than ever before, and totally in love with my thighs. I'm not sure when the shift happened, but I know it was somewhere on the journey to the powerful lift-ups in the practice that I finally learned how to believe in myself. Now, when I look back at old pictures of myself, I don't see the same things I did then. I see a beautiful girl who just never believed in her own beauty.

Through the subtlety of the inner body, you feel your true nature and learn to have faith in yourself. The faith cultivated through yoga is based in direct experience. Only by directly perceiving the self within is it possible to have faith in that self. Eschew external standards and judgments, and be solid in your authenticity. Know without a doubt what it means to truly trust yourself. Have faith that you are okay, believe that you are whole and complete, and finally recognize that you are strong enough and worthy of love. You are beautiful and whole and divinely created. Look for a little voice that says, *Maybe I can be strong too.* Decide to believe in yourself and never give up.

HOMEWORK

1. Question. Today ask yourself, *What do I believe in? What do I have faith in?* You might believe in the practice; you might believe in love; eventually you might be brave enough to believe in the quiet voice of wisdom in your heart. What will it take for you to believe in yourself and in the practice? Some people believe without any evidence. Others need hard proof and lots of experience.

2. Have faith in your body. Celebrate at least one key point about your body. Reflect on one major accomplishment it has allowed you to attain. Perhaps you have given birth or completed a marathon or a challenging hike. Or perhaps you have been practicing yoga every day for the last several years. Whatever your physical accomplishment, recognize that your body is a divine gift and celebrate your faith in it.

3. Believe. Look in the mirror and say these words aloud to yourself: "I believe I am healed. I believe I am worthy of love. I believe I am enough. I believe in me."

PRACTICE

1. *Malasana*—Garland Pose

While every yoga pose has the opportunity to teach you how to be faithful and believe in yourself, Malasana represents the small seed of faith that is planted in your heart.

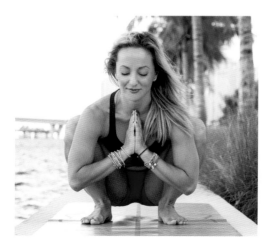

Start off in a squatting position. Open your knees as you send your torso forward between your legs. Drop your head and chest while keeping your shins tucked with your upper arms. Draw your thighs close to your shoulders, and press your shoulders back into your thighs. Place your hands in prayer position. Tuck your tailbone and keep your lower belly drawn in deeply. Gaze at the tip of your nose or close your eyes. Stay here for five breaths, then release.

2. *Pasasana*—Noose Pose

Pasasana is the first pose of the traditional Ashtanga Yoga Intermediate Series.

Start off in a squatting position with your feet together; use a towel or wedge under your heels if they do not reach the ground. Inhale to create space behind your pubic bone; exhale to fold your torso toward the left side. Drop your right shoulder under your left knee. Rotate your right shoulder inward as you wrap your right elbow around both shins. Inhale as you lift your left arm and reach around your back for your right hand. Clasp your hands together on the upper portion of your right thigh. Stay here for five breaths. Come back to center and repeat on the left side.

If you cannot bind your hands, then simply reach around and bring your hands as close together as possible. The key element of faith in Pasasana comes when you reach your hands toward each other. Since you are literally reaching blindly and have no way to see where your hands are, you will need to feel your way with your body and trust that the bind will one day be possible. As both a teacher and a student, I have seen that the hands are often much closer together than you might initially think. With faith and consistent practice, this twist will become possible.

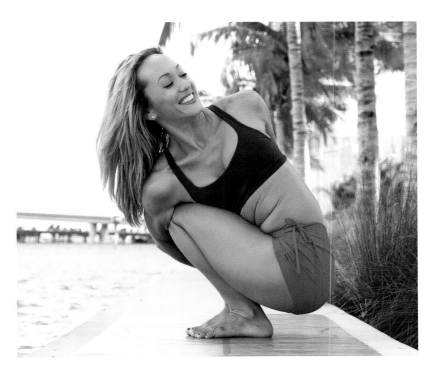

3. *Parsva Bakasana*—Side Crane Pose

This pose is often linked with Pasasana. In fact, you could think about this as a lifted version of the twist. Twisting arm balances rely on the shoulders for foundation and then articulate the twist throughout the spine and hips.

Start off in a squatting position and fold your torso to the left side, or continue directly from the first side of Pasasana. Place your hands on the ground, shoulder-width apart, and allow your elbows to bend slightly. Stack your knees as close to your right shoulder as possible. Lean forward and come onto the tips of your toes. Engage your lower abdominal muscles, activate your internal oblique muscles, and draw in your lower ribs. Inhale as you lift by sending your body forward onto your arms. Send your hips up and toward the right side while gluing your thighs together. Straighten your arms as much as possible. Stay here for five breaths. Come down and repeat on the other side.

The "lift up" moment in Parsva Bakasana requires a great leap of faith into the strength of your shoulders. It may feel like you cannot suspend yourself off to the side like this. But over time, you will develop trust in yourself and your body.

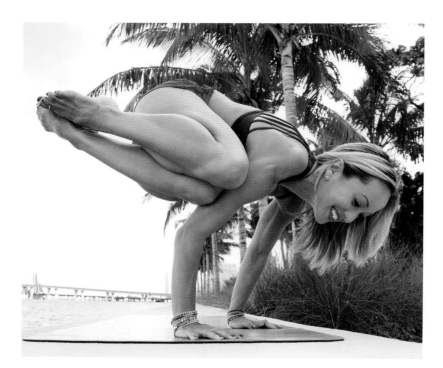

4. *Laghuvajrasana*—Little Thunderbolt Pose

Many students leave this pose feeling defeated. While the name of the pose is often translated as Little Thunderbolt, I like to think of it as the Little Thunderbolt That Could. You will need to be vigilant against doubt, indecision, and weakness of body and mind if you are to succeed in Laghuvajrasana. The Little Thunderbolt must be internalized as a show of inner strength.

Start off in a kneeling position. Inhale as you rise up on your knees, create maximum space between your ribs and hips, and begin to arch your spine. Exhale as you send your hips forward and drop your hands down to your ankles. Grab hold of your ankles by placing your thumbs on the insides of your ankles and your fingers on the outsides. Press firmly into the heels of your hands. Continue the exhalation as you bend your knees and send your body out long to rest the top of your head on the ground. Keep your arms straight and your hands around your ankles to fully enter Laghuvajrasana. Stay here for five breaths.

Going down is usually not the problem. It's once you're down that you may feel totally stuck. This is where you need faith. When you feel blocked, don't immediately give up. Instead, follow your breath, feel your hips, and stick to the technique. Send your hips forward, firm your quadriceps, rotate your hips inward, and push (don't pull!) with your arms. Leave your head back and just keep sending your hips forward to come up. If you can't exit the pose this way, then stay in it for fifteen breaths, applying the technique and building faith that one day you will be able to come up. Most important, leave the pose with a sense of faith in yourself—never leave feeling defeated.

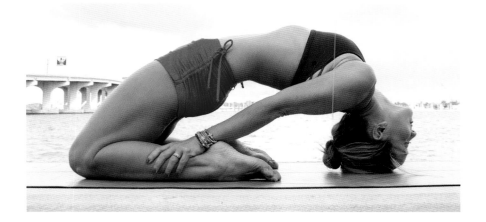

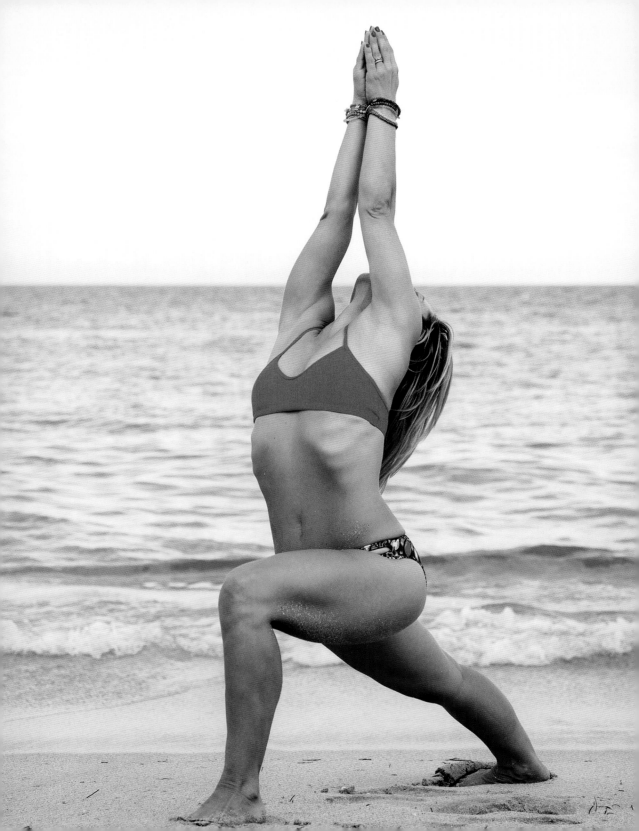

Being Your Own Hero
Vira

Virabhadrasana A and B (Warrior Pose I and II) are named after a mythic warrior who was created out of a lock of hair from the Hindu deity Shiva. In need of a warrior to avenge the death of his wife, Shiva grew angry and threw one of his dreadlocks down to earth. When it landed, Virabhadra was formed in the shape of Virabhadrasana A, holding a sword above his head. Upon landing with his legs in the familiar pose, he then opened his arms, switched his gaze forward, and took aim in Virabhadrasana B. So the actual shape of the pose is based on the warrior's mythic stance. Although his first task was one of vengeance, Virabhadra later became known as a symbol of dharma, the notion that eventually good wins out over evil. The transformation from the personalized struggles of the ego to the socially conscious stance of justice mirrors the journey of most yoga practitioners; we start the journey consumed by personal struggle and hurt only to find purpose and meaning through the practice.

Today's yogi assignment is *vira*, the hero. Part of the journey of yoga is about becoming the hero of your own life story. Being a yogi is a spiritual journey, and you carry the mantle of inner truth into the world. As a yogi, you are asked to do much more than stretch and bend your body; you are asked to make the world a more peaceful place.

Shri K. Pattabhi Jois would often recommend that students read the great epic story of the Bhagavad Gita as inspiration for their practice. Arjuna, the warrior prince and hero of the story, seeks the counsel of Krishna, who is an incarnation of God. The battle that takes place in the Gita, as described in Day One, is not just a physical one; it is a metaphor for the inner fight. Arjuna is both the perfect yogi and a mighty warrior. He is humble, kindhearted, and teachable. Yet he is strong and proficient with his weaponry. He seeks not only victory but a clear conscience and a righteous relationship with God. He reminds us that we must make a choice each day, and perhaps even each moment, to orient the mind toward the world within instead of the temptations and distractions of the external world.

Guruji recommended that his students read the Gita because our lives reflect the battle in this book more closely than they do the lofty stories of yogis in caves. We are constantly tempted, yet we must strive to be humble and kind and focused on completing the task at hand. Essentially we must become like Arjuna in our daily lives—filled simultaneously with the strength and magnificence of a warrior prince and the peace and sanctity of a spiritual aspirant. To be a yogi is to be strong enough to contain these seemingly opposite concepts in our hearts.

The yoga practice is a hero's journey that leads you to the center of yourself. Rather than traveling to distant lands, the spiritual journey happens in the inner body. Your body is the terra firma for exploration. Instead of perfecting the use of a weapon, you attain mastery over your sense organs and have the power to control the mind. Controlling the mind means you can recast yourself in the hero's role and change your inner dialogue from weakness to grace and strength. You may choose to take on a cause and fight for social justice. Or you may simply choose to commit yourself to acting and speaking out of love for yourself, others, and your community. Once you embody the brave heart of the yogi, every action flows from a place of deep inner resolution, and you will be a force of healing in the world.

HOMEWORK **1. Practice humility.** Close your eyes. Drop the mind into the inner body and feel the space under your skin. Yoga is not a competition; it is a path of awakening. It is a sacred space of reverence that must be approached with humility. Recognize that everything is really a gift. We don't own anything that matters. Our breath, our lives, our bodies are all divine gifts. There is no copyright on love, joy, forgiveness, or peace. We work and strive, but only by grace do we attain anything. When people tell me they have experienced transformation and healing in class with me, I know it's not me. Yoga is a gift, a sacred practice of inner realization. All the power, healing, and grace come from God. Humility comes when you recognize this basic truth with respect and reverence. Trust the divine plan for your life, humbly ask for help, and let yourself be guided beyond your wildest dreams. Be humble, be kind, be a yogi in the world.

2. Find *virya*. Translated as "energy, enthusiasm, and vigor," virya is what the hero needs to complete the journey. Cultivate enthusiasm for yoga practice, and it will ignite your life! Inspiration is the source of virya, the spiritual strength that it takes to walk the path of yoga. It can be hard to motivate yourself to get on your mat in the morning when you want to sleep in and stay out late at night. Finding inspiration to live more peacefully is the heart of the spiritual practice. Take a few moments to reconnect with your inspiration to practice. Think about your teacher or watch an inspiring yoga video. When you get on your mat today, cultivate a can-do attitude that willingly takes on the challenge of the inner work regardless of how deeply you get into the physical poses of the practice.

3. Be your own hero. Is there a place in your life where you feel victimized? How can you change your perspective and become your own hero? Instead of waiting for external circumstances to change, begin to change the story line of your life by thinking different thoughts, feeling different feelings, and engaging in different actions.

1. *Virabhadrasana A*—Warrior I Pose

The two most common versions of Virabhadrasana are traditionally done in succession. Linking Virabhadrasana A and B together increases the strength and stamina required for the poses and encourages the inner hero's journey. This pose is usually entered from Adho Mukha Svanasana. Inhale as you step your left foot forward and take a wide stance, leaving approximately one leg-length between your feet. This distance is adjustable based on your height, leg length, and level of flexibility. Plant your right heel on the ground and rotate your right hip outward about forty-five degrees. Align your left heel with your right arch. Press firmly into the bases of your big toes, bases of your little toes, and your heels. Sink down into your legs until your left thigh is parallel to the ground. Stack your torso directly on top of your hips. Suck in your lower belly and lift your spine along the central axis. Put hands in prayer position. Raise your arms in line with your torso, straighten your elbows, and gaze up at your thumbs.

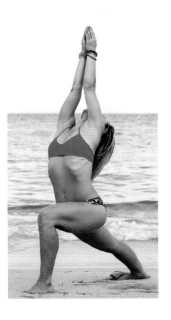

Be brave in the midst of any burning sensations along your thighs or other areas of muscular exhaustion. Stay here for five breaths, then repeat on the right side.

2. *Virabhadrasana B*—Warrior II Pose

Continuing directly from Virabhadrasana A on the left side, open your arms and spread your shoulders apart. Send your right hip back to open the groin and inner thigh. Maintain the strength and stability of your legs and the spaciousness between your ribs and hips. Equalize your sitting bones. Reach your arms equally out toward your feet. Gaze at the fingertips of your left hand. Stay here for five breaths, then repeat on the right side. After five breaths on the right side, place your hands on the ground and step back to Chaturanga Dandasana.

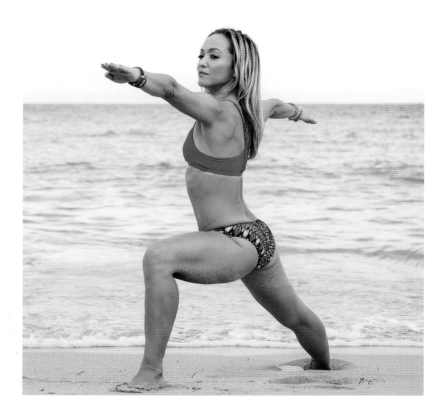

3. *Viparita Virabhadrasana*—Reverse Warrior Pose

Whereas Virabhadrasana A and B are traditionally linked together, Virabhadrasana is a slightly more advanced pose and is better to practice on its own. Start in Adho Mukha Svanasana. Inhale and set up for a stable Virabhadrasana A, with your right leg forward. If you feel any restriction in this foundational pose, do not proceed further. If you are ready to proceed, reach your left hand back toward your left knee, gently activating and encouraging a spinal extension. Roll your left shoulder forward into an internal rotation and firm the muscles around your shoulder girdle. Avoid hinging back or twisting too much to the left. Stabilize your left leg, engage your quadriceps, and keep as much space as possible between your ribs and hips. Inhale and reach your right arm back by deepening the external rotation of your shoulder. Roll your armpit toward your chin, and when you feel comfortable, allow your neck to drop back gently. Gaze either at the fingertips of your right hand or back toward your left foot. Stay here for five breaths. Gently inhale and return to Virabhadrasana A. Exhale as you place your hands on the ground and step back to Chaturanga Dandasana. Inhale as you move forward to Urdhva Mukha Svanasana, exhale and move back to Adho Mukha Svanasana. Inhale, step forward with your left foot, and repeat the sequence.

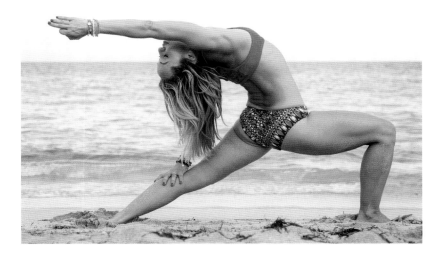

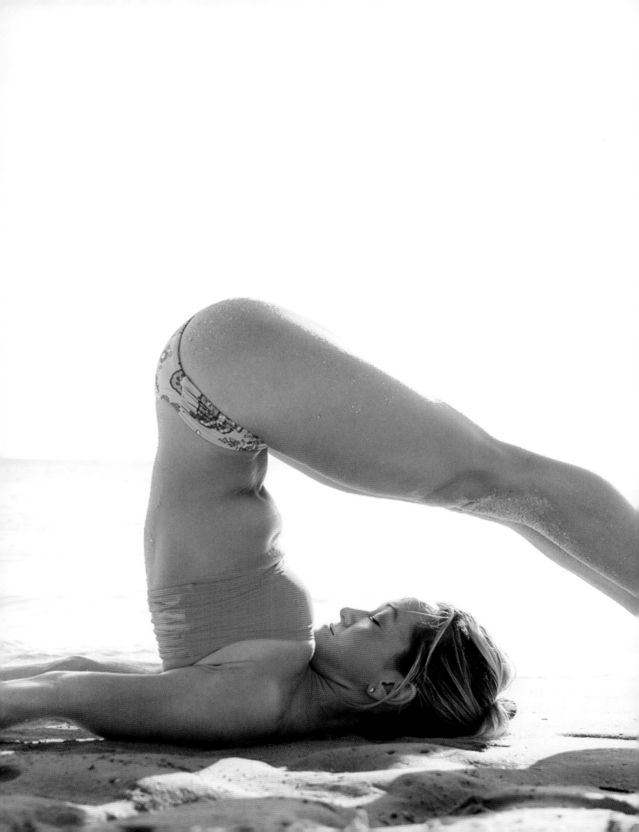

Day 15 | Peace
Shanti

used to plan everything far in advance, stressing out about the small details on everything from a shopping list to my progress in asana. I set goals for my life and then nearly killed myself trying to attain them. I got anxious when life didn't unfold according to my schedule. When I first started my practice, I used to feel like I had to give 150 percent every single time in every single breath or else I would be slacking off. When someone told me not to try so hard, I thought she was nuts. While a certain degree of planning and effort is healthy and necessary, my overplanning and obsessing about the future stemmed from a lack of trust. My need to control the outcome of everything was rooted in an inherent mistrust of the universe—and ultimately, myself. It also gave me tunnel vision, which cut me off from experiencing the peace of the present moment.

One day, after nearly ten years of practice, I was in the middle of a ten-day meditation retreat and got this brilliant idea to relax and see what happened. And you know what? It was amazing! As soon as I started to let go of all that extra effort, my heart and mind began to open up to receive things that were bigger than I could have imagined. When I stopped trying to bend the world to my will, I started to experience the magic of Divine will. It sounds simple, but learning to relax was not easy for me. It is like finding the sweet spot between just the right amount of effort and surrender, the perfect mix of strength and grace.

Patanjali says in Yoga Sutra 2.47 that after the firm posture of asana is established, we should relax all unnecessary effort and meditate on the infinite. Letting go of the need to control recognizes that thinking you can control anything is a delusion of the ego. Try to bend someone to your will, and it always goes wrong. Try to bend the world to your will, and it will fight back. But relax, surrender, and let it all go, and you will experience the freedom that is the heart of yoga.

Today's yogi assignment is *shanti*, meaning "peace." This will be a hard lesson for all you type A planners and control freaks like me. Personally, I could not accept surrendering my control without the corollary amount of faith. First, I learned to have faith in my teacher, Shri K. Pattabhi Jois. When I first met him in India as a newbie Ashtanga Yoga practitioner, he told me, "Shanti is coming, no problem." I heard that as a promise he made to me, and I believed in it because I believed in him. I diligently kept practicing, and after many years, I can verify that the promise of shanti holds true. This practice slowly shifts the arc of your life toward peace. I didn't believe I could live a more peaceful life, but Guruji saw it as just a matter of time.

Peace isn't a mythical realm on a lotus flower. In yoga, it's an action and a choice. It's not like I never worry or stress out anymore. Instead, when I find myself fretting, I ask for that burden to be lifted off my heart. Beyond belief in my teacher, yoga has given me a direct experience of the Divine spirit within me. I needed to believe in a Higher Power, a force whose magnificence and boundless compassion I could trust to take care of the direction of my life so I could fully experience peace of mind. No amount of worrying or stressing is going to change any situation. Only with faith in the basic goodness of the universe can you find peace.

Shanti is perhaps best understood as a place to rest your heart and mind. I have found rest in a life lived in communion with spirit. And so can you, just by doing this practice over many years. The promise of the practice is that shanti will come for you too, no problem!

HOMEWORK **1. Release control.** Ask yourself what you're trying to control in your life, what you're holding on to tightly, and where that impulse comes from. You might be holding on to old emotions, detailed plans, or perfectionism. Whatever it is most likely comes from fear and insecurity. Identify one thing you can relax about today, and let it go. Trust in the purity of your true self; relax, soften, and just be. Pause and see how you feel.

2. Practice Divine stress relief. Tune in today and see what your biggest worry or stress is. Take a few moments to calm the mind through cultivating a meditative state. Then ask for that burden to be lifted from your heart and turn it over to God or a force greater than yourself.

Recognize that no amount of worrying will make any difference, and surrender your will to this greater force with the full faith and trust that what is meant to happen will happen and that everything is working for your greater good. Don't stop working; just stop stressing.

3. Try the no-planning experiment. Set aside one day this week that you don't plan. Go with the flow and see where life leads you. At the end of the day, reflect on the unexpected surprises that were only possible because you didn't plan them. Use this as empirical proof that things work out just fine, if not better, when you don't try to arrange every little detail of your life.

1. *Anjaneyasana*—Low Lunge

This crescent lunge is named after Hanuman, the monkey deity, whose pose (Hanumanasana) is the full split. Regular practice of Anjaneyasana will indeed open your hips and prepare the way for a full split. However, when you begin working toward the deep hip and back extension required for the splits, it is easy to become frustrated. Instead, remain peaceful, and use Anjaneyasana to cultivate an attitude of inner tranquility.

Start in Adho Mukha Svanasana. Step your left foot forward; bend your right knee and place it on the ground. Square your hips forward. Leave approximately on leg-length between your left heel and the toes of your right foot. This distance is adjustable based on your height, leg length, and level of flexibility. Your right hip should already be in an extended position to start the pose. If you notice your left knee moving past your toes, step your left foot forward to make more space. Inhale as you lift your torso and stack your body along the center line. Exhale and place your hands in prayer position to enter stage one.

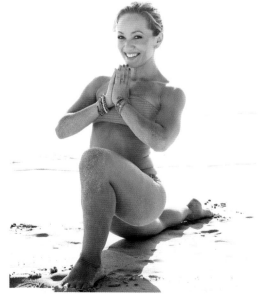

PEACE SHANTI

105

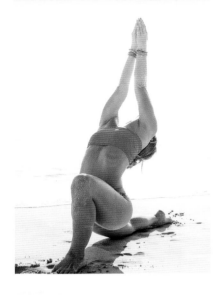

Inhale as you raise your arms straight up and maximize the space between your ribs and hips. Stay here if you feel you have reached your limit. If possible, extend your arms back and over your head, gazing toward either your fingertips or your right heel to enter the full expression of Anjaneyasana. Stay here for five breaths. Inhale as you slowly bring your hands back to stage one. Exhale, place your hands on the ground, and step back to Chaturanga Dandasana. Repeat on the other side.

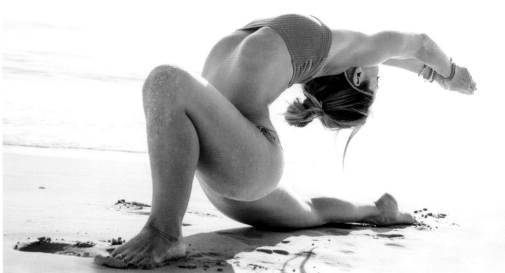

2. *Urdhva Hasta Hanumanasana*—Handstand Splits

Balance in handstand comes from a calm and peaceful mind. If you disturb the balance of your mind while attempting the pose, you will essentially block your body from achieving it.

Start in Adho Mukha Svanasana and walk your feet half the distance to your hands. Stabilize your shoulder girdle and prepare your arms to receive the weight of your body. Step your right foot forward while bending your knees, press firmly into your arms, and inhale as your left leg floats up. Shift your hips onto the foundation of your arms.

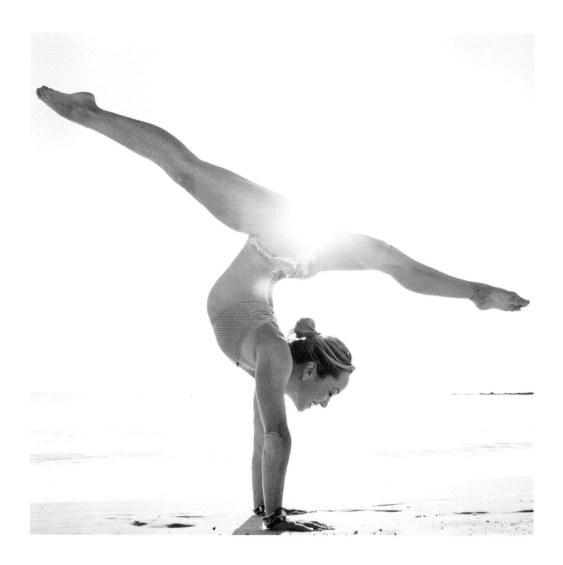

Think of stepping your body weight onto your arms instead of fling-
ing yourself up. Stack your shoulders over your palms. Reach forward
with your left leg to open your thighs into the fullest expression of the
Handstand Split that is accessible to you. Gaze between your hands to
avoid overarching your spine. Stay here for five breaths and then slowly
come down. Repeat, reaching forward with your right leg this time.

   If you are not able to achieve balance on the left side, try three
times with a peaceful attitude of tolerance and patience, then try on
the other side.

3. *Halasana/Karnapidasana*—Plow Pose/Ear Pressure Pose

These two poses are part of the traditional Ashtanga Yoga Closing Series and offer the chance to turn the mind inward and integrate a peaceful attitude. Halasana and Karnapidasana are best done in succession. If you have worked with deep spinal extensions, these two poses will help your body and mind retain a sense of peace.

You can enter these poses directly from Salami Sarvangasana (Shoulderstand) or lift up from a reclining position. If you are starting from a supine position, then inhale and lift your hips while keeping your legs close into your torso until you roll all the way over and your feet touch the floor over the top of your head. Roll your shoulders under your body and actively press your shoulders down to create space behind your neck. Interlock your fingers and straighten your arms. Align your feet, point your toes, and slide the tops of your feet toward the ground to enter Halasana. Straighten your spine and lift your sitting bones to replicate the sensation of Dandasana, and stay here for eight to ten breaths.

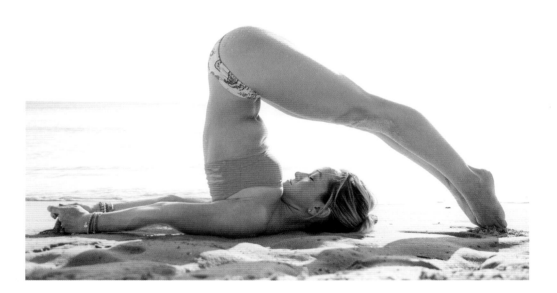

For Karnapidasana, round your back, tuck your tailbone, and squeeze your knees down toward your ears to accentuate the sensation of compressing the torso. Stay here for another eight to ten breaths.

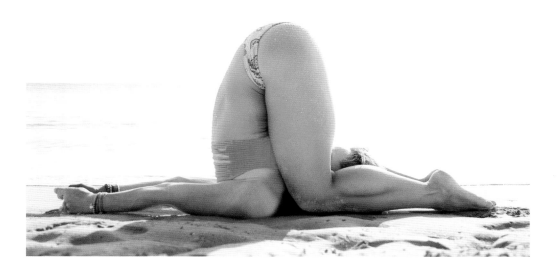

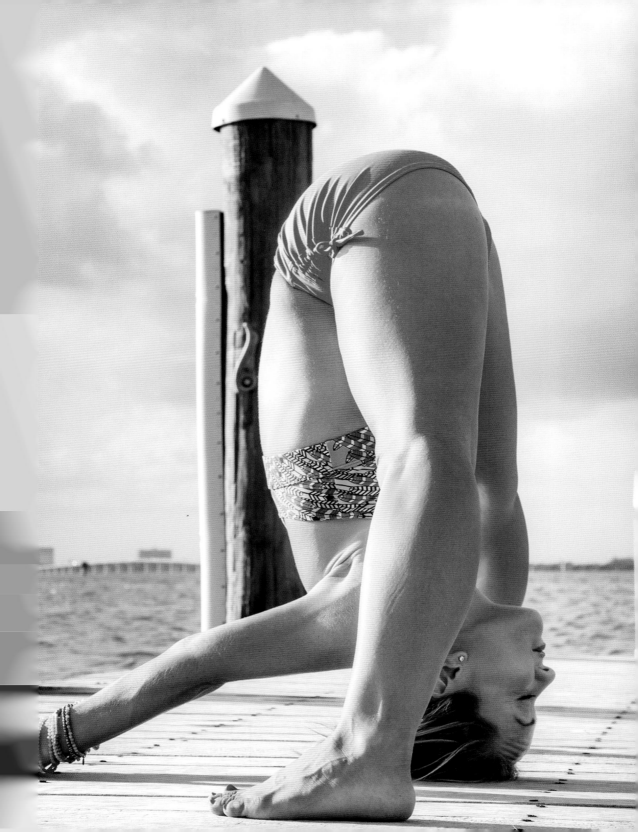

Forgiveness
Ksama

There is a spring festival in India called Holi, when people throw rainbow powder all over the place. I remember waking up in Mysore to an explosion of multicolored cows and people's faces spattered with the brilliance of a carnival. Celebrated on the vernal equinox, this festival of love is traditionally a day of forgiveness and a time to heal ruptured relationships. Forgiveness is an essential lesson on the journey of yoga; it's as freeing as a grand celebration and leads the practitioner to a happier life.

Today's yogi assignment is forgiveness (*ksama*). This message of reconciliation is an important step in accepting yourself and your life in all their extraordinary imperfections; a humble request to be loved as you are and to love your world as it is. Ask yourself if you are holding on to any anger, resentment, or feelings of victimization, and see if you are ready to let them go with the simple and powerful act of forgiveness. Trust is a gift that, after it has been abused or taken for granted, must be earned again. By granting or asking for forgiveness, you open a channel into the receptive, soft heart that is full of love.

When you decide to take on yoga as a sincere and spiritual practice, you take a vow in your heart to live a more peaceful life. You share a commitment with yogis all over the world to live a dharmic life, aligned with yogic moral and ethical guidelines. Yet despite our best efforts, we make mistakes. Regardless of our commitment to do good, we will inadvertently hurt someone or take action that leads to suffering. While we strive to be peaceful in every moment, not one among us is totally free from emotional baggage.

From a traditional perspective, the yogi-as-spiritual-seeker cultivates forgiveness for wrongs done to him or her out of a desire to be free from any remaining negative thoughts. Forgiveness is an act of self-love and self-affirmation that acknowledges that holding on to bitterness only further damages oneself. Reconciling with the person who committed the wrong is secondary to the yogi's personal act of forgiveness. The power of forgiveness in its highest state allows us to remain equanimous, free from anger or animosity, and strong enough to never play the victim. The strength it takes to put this into action is perhaps the greatest test on the yogi's path. How many times must you forgive? As many times as you have been wronged. This requires great strength and faith.

When I first started my practice, I held myself so strictly to what I perceived to be the moral code for living the yogi's life that I was surely doomed to fail. I performed my daily asana ritual with extreme devotion and determination. I changed my diet to follow strict raw vegan guidelines, gave up all makeup, and wore only organic cotton clothes. But this was simply unsustainable. When I failed to live up to my own high standards on or off the yoga mat, I mentally beat myself up. I felt like I wasn't good enough and that I had to work hard to prove my worthiness. If I missed a day of intensive practice, used a little eyeliner, or ate a cupcake, I had yogi's guilt over it. After I had been practicing for about ten years, I remember feeling really down about myself because I wasn't further along the asana road or the road to spiritual liberation. This may sound completely ridiculous, but I literally had to forgive myself because I wasn't already enlightened and my handstands weren't as good as I wanted them to be. I had to accept and love myself as I was, with whatever strength, peace, and enlightenment I had been able to experience.

Since then, as a teacher, I have often found that the more diligent and sincere students are, the harder they are on themselves. Instead of using the practice to try to "fix" yourself and "prove" that you are good enough, use it as a place where you experience the truth of who you are. There is a spirit within each of us. Your sincere desire to live a more peaceful life is the key that unlocks the door to freedom. Forgive yourself and begin the journey today. Forgive others and set them free. Ask for forgiveness and work to win back trust. We all carry the scars of painful and traumatic experiences to varying degrees. We all carry the weight of things we have done for which we feel remorse, regret, or embarrassment. We can only truly heal through forgiveness. Practice is defined by the steady commitment to get on your mat every day; a humble heart that is willing to practice through good and bad days; a tenacious spirit; a clear and focused mind; a fire of motivation that illuminates the next step on the inner path; and a compassionate worldview filled with patience, forgiveness, peace, and joy.

1. Forgive someone. Who can you forgive today to clear your past? Don't wait for people to say they're sorry before you let go of the bitterness in your heart. Prepare yourself to receive apologies you may never get, and let go of the emotional baggage stored in your own heart today.

2. Forgive yourself. Is it yourself that you need to forgive? Stop beating yourself up for yesterday's mistakes or your perceived shortcomings. Let your past experience make you wise and humble. Stop self-denigrating behavior. Forgive yourself and let it go.

3. Ask for forgiveness. Is there someone you have hurt knowingly or unknowingly from whom you must ask forgiveness? With a humble heart, free of expectation, offer your apology to free yourself, but don't get upset if the person doesn't accept it or welcome you with open arms.

1. *Prasarita Padottanasana C*—Wide-Legged Forward Bend C PRACTICE

Start in Samasthiti. Inhale and step your feet about one leg-length apart. This distance is adjustable based on height, leg length, and level of flexibility. Spread your arms out to the sides. Exhale as you clasp your hands together behind your back, interlace your fingers, and straighten your arms. Inhale again, creating space in your lower belly. Exhale as you fold forward. Pivot through your hip joints, suck in your belly, and relax your shoulders down toward the ground. Rotate your shoulders inward, and breathe deeply to enter Prasarita Padottanasana C. The full pose means the top of your head is on the ground between your feet and your hands reach the ground in front of you. Avoid pulling or forcing your hands toward the ground; instead, surrender, relax, and lengthen. Feel the inner body. Stay here for five breaths.

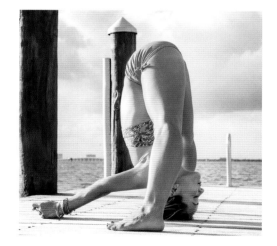

FORGIVENESS KSAMA

Practice being gentle with yourself, and forgive yourself for any tightness. Accept your body as it is, and just be with your breath. Inhale as you come up, drawing your pubic bone forward to elevate your trunk. Exhale and settle your hands at your waist.

2. *Supta Padangusthasana*—Reclining Hand-to-Big-Toe Pose

Start off in a supine position. Straighten your legs, suck in your belly, draw your thighs together, point your toes, and place your hands on the tops of your hips. Stabilize your hips and firm your pelvic floor. Inhale as you lift your right leg and hold on to the right foot with your right hand. Exhale as you lift your head toward your knee and elevate your trunk. Firm your left quadricep and root down through your left heel. Stay here for five breaths.

Inhale as you settle your head back toward the ground. Exhale and roll your right leg out to the side. Allow the movement to happen by rotating your right hip joint outward. Stabilize the left side of your pelvis, and avoid hiking your left hip in an attempt to place your right foot on the ground. Instead, let the placement of your right foot be determined by the level of external rotation facilitated by your hip joint. Maintain a calm, equanimous, and gentle attitude toward your body. Stay here for another five breaths.

Inhale and roll through your right hip joint to bring your right leg back to center. Exhale as you again lift your head toward your knee and elevate your trunk. Inhale and lower your head back to the ground. Exhale as you release and lower your right leg. Repeat on the left side.

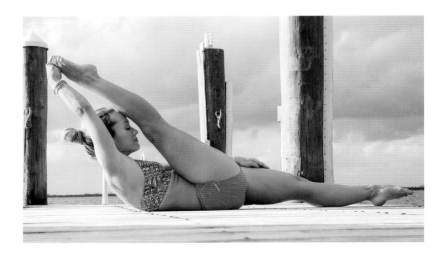

3. *Salami Sarvangasana*—Shoulderstand

Sarvangasana is actually translated as "all-limbs pose" and activates all the limbs of the body.

Start off in a supine position, and inhale as you lift your legs. First bring your legs to a ninety-degree angle with the floor. Then continue lifting by engaging your pelvic floor until your hips are stacked on top of your shoulders. Point your toes, and orient your torso toward the vertical axis to come all the way up into Sarvangasana. Place your flattened hands on your lower back, and close your fingers. Draw your lower ribs in and activate your quadriceps. Press your shoulders into the ground as you rotate them inward. Your elbows should be aligned with your shoulders. Rest your chin on your sternum, and keep the back of your neck off the ground. Stay here for ten to fifteen breaths. Release your hands, and slowly pivot down through your hip joints. Focus on turning your attention inward with a humble heart.

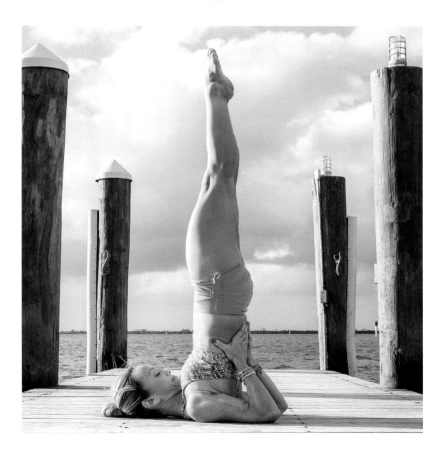

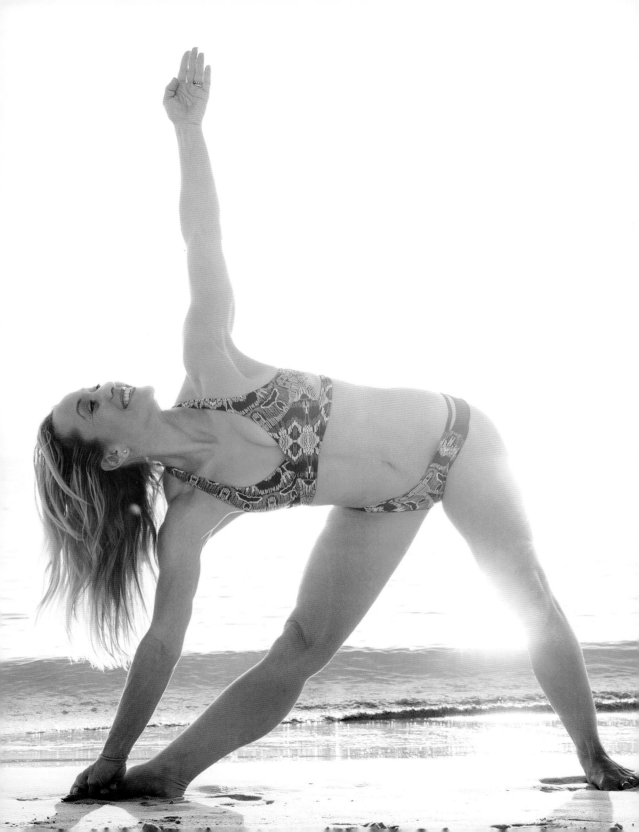

Ignorance
Avidya

Knowledge is power, but limited knowledge can be a trap. What you think you "know" may in fact be only part of the whole story. It can also be hard to navigate the murky territory between knowledge and judgment. The only thing I definitely know is that I will never actually have all the answers, see the full picture, and have the omniscience to know it all, all the time, every time.

Today's yogi assignment is ignorance (*avidya*). Avidya is the lack of knowledge of the true self, which is considered to be the root of all suffering—and the main obstacle on the spiritual path. Avidya can also manifest as ignorance, the unwillingness to see, admit, or recognize the truth when it is revealed to you. Sometimes we hold on to knowledge in the effort to build up a false sense of self, to be "somebody" in the eyes of the world.

Patanjali states in Yoga Sutra 1.7 that there are three types of epistemological paradigms for the acquisition of knowledge. The first is *agama*, meaning devotional knowledge or information that you accept based on faith in the source. This includes information you receive from a trusted source like your teacher or your parents, as well as information you glean from sacred texts. The second is *anumana*, or logical knowledge gained from inference, deduction, and the faculties of reason. This is information that makes sense to you. The third is *pratyaksa*, experiential knowledge that understands something to be true because it has been directly perceived. This empirical proof standard is considered the highest form of knowledge in yoga philosophy because it has the power to change your view. Knowledge based in direct experience may not always make sense to you, but because you have experienced it, you accept it. Logic is limited by our human faculties and bound by the limits of our mind. Devotion is often tied up with our emotions. But direct experience has the potential to shift your worldview.

Yoga practice is based on the premise that only the knowledge you have experienced to be true puts you on firm ground. All other knowledge shifts more easily and is not considered stable. By heightening your powers of direct perception, yoga offers you a laboratory in which to test your experience and knowledge. First, you directly feel your muscles, then the subtler energy shifts, then the inner body, then the immutable spirit within, and finally the Divine.

Spiritual self-inquiry traditionally takes the form of either studying the sacred texts of the spiritual path like the Yoga Sutras, the Bible, or the Dhammapada or a study of the true self, a sincere effort directed at the highest truth within, and a concentrated discipline directed at the direct experience of Divine wisdom. If you already feel like you have all the answers, knowledge, and wisdom, then there is no space for the light of higher awareness to seep in. Only by admitting with humility that you need to study, learn, and devote yourself to the spiritual path will you find the hidden keys to true self-knowledge.

Yoga is about humility and surrender. Admitting that you don't know something is the first step on the journey of knowledge. In many ways, the humility to admit what we don't know is the basic requirement for a student of yoga. As a yoga teacher, there are numerous times when a student asks me a question and I simply don't know the answer. Rather than trying to fake it, I just say that I don't know. If it's important or I can find the answer, then I will research and report back. But sometimes I don't know the answer, and I know I won't be able to find it. And that's okay. Admitting that you don't know is not a sign of weakness; it's a sign of self-assurance. It also sets you free. Yoga teachers have a responsibility to be vigilant in recognizing the limitations of their own knowledge. Remembering that we are all, first and foremost, students engaged in the discovery of the true self keeps us humble and on the right path.

The entire teaching of yoga is built on the premise that we suffer because we are confused about who we really are. Once we directly experience the truth of who we are, the root ignorance is removed and we are free. All yoga practitioners seek deeper experiences of the truth to reach deeper levels of freedom until the ultimate truth of the spirit is revealed, along with the ultimate experience of freedom. The lack of knowledge of the true self is considered to be the root obstacle, the *mula klesha* from which all other obstacles spring. If the root of the tree of suffering is removed, then all its fruits will also be removed. First, yoga teaches you how to know your body and mind from the inside out.

Then it guides you into the realms of subtler inner experience. Finally, it provides a bridge to let you directly perceive the Divine. I believe it is possible for every single person to have a transcendent experience of the highest self within and that those moments of intimate connection with God are what life is really about.

Today, rest in the purity of your true self and say the words "I don't know." Not knowing doesn't make you any less of a person. Realizing that you don't have to have all the answers is like letting a huge burden fall off your shoulders. Instead of trying to prove yourself, just *be* yourself.

HOMEWORK

1. Imagine a knowledge diagram. State three examples of the following two types of knowledge: what you know and what you don't know. For example, what you know could be how to read; what you don't know could be how it feels to walk on the moon. Then contemplate the vast, infinite expanse of what you don't know you don't know.

2. Identify knowledge types. List two pieces of information that you accept based on the three knowledge paradigms presented in yoga (devotional, rational, and experiential).

3. Admit your ignorance. Look for an opportunity to say the words "I don't know" today in response to a question. If you need to research the answer, then admit what you do not know and go study. If you do not need to know the answer, then simply admit your limitations and let that set you free.

PRACTICE

1. *Trikonasana*—Triangle Pose

While Trikonasana is often seen as a relatively simple pose, if you approach it with a keen sensitivity to the inner body, it can transform your relationship with your hip joints and pelvic floor. Instead of focusing on perfect physical or aesthetic form, think of this pose as a chance to discover your hip joint from the inside out. Dive down into your pelvis and feel your way through to the subtler sensations within the darkness of the inner world.

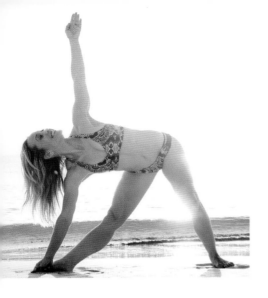

Start in Samasthiti. Inhale as you step out to the right, leaving a distance just shorter than one leg-length between your feet. This distance is adjustable based on your height, leg length, and level of flexibility. Externally rotate your right hip joint, and align your right heel with your left arch. Extend your arms out to the sides as far as possible at shoulder height, and create space in the inner body by sucking in your belly and lifting your ribs away from your hips along the center line. Exhale as you fold into your right hip joint and reach your right hand down toward your right big toe; your left arm points up to the sky. If possible, wrap your fingers around your big toe and pull upward to keep your shoulders active. If you cannot reach your toes, then allow your hand to rest along your shin. Gaze up toward the fingertips of your left hand. Draw your lower ribs and navel in toward your spine. Stay here for five breaths. Inhale as you come up. Repeat on the left side.

2. Ardha Baddha Padmottanasana— Half-Bound Lotus Standing Forward Fold

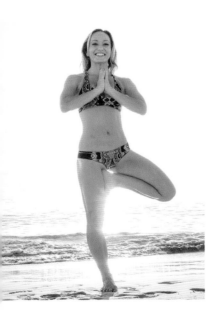

To enter any of the lotus poses, you need a deep knowledge of the inner space of your hips and knees. Ardha Baddha Padmottanasana combines an external rotation of the hips with a deep forward fold. More than intellectual understanding, you need to feel your hips and knees at each step of entering this pose to determine how far to proceed. Without the inner body knowledge provided through sensation and awareness, it is unfortunately rather easy to push too hard and create injury instead of awakening.

Start off in Samasthiti. Inhale as you glide your left foot into Vrksasana (Tree Pose). You should continue only if your left knee feels good and your left hip feels open. When you are ready, slide your left foot into Half Lotus. Draw the instep of your left foot toward your right hip crease. Align your left foot toward the outer edge of your navel on the right side. Reach your left hand around your back and wrap your fingers around your left foot. If you cannot reach your foot, then simply hold your right elbow. Gaze downward, and if your left knee feels good, exhale and fold

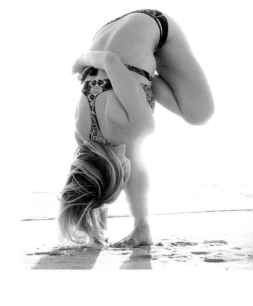

forward. Lift your lower belly in deeply and reach your lower abdominal muscles away from your left foot. Align your right hand with your right foot, and reach your chin toward your right shin. If your knee does not feel comfortable, do not *under any circumstances* attempt to fold forward. If you lose your balance, you can place both hands on the ground for greater control. Gaze forward toward your right toes. Stay here for five breaths.

Keep your subnavel drawn in toward your spine and stabilize your standing leg. Inhale and send your chest forward to come up partway; exhale to stabilize. Inhale as you come up to standing and release your left foot. Return to Samasthiti. Repeat on the right side.

3. *Dandasana*—Staff Pose

Think of Dandasana as the seated version of Samasthiti. It is a seated pose that maintains an orientation toward the center line and sets the baseline from which all other seated poses originate. Whenever you jump through to seated from Adho Mukha Svanasana, you are advised to land in Dandasana for a moment to collect and orient your body to the center line before moving into the next pose.

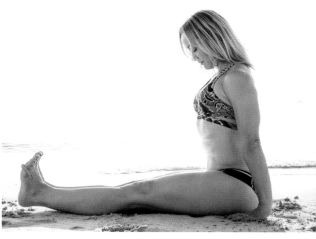

Start off in a seated position with your legs straight out. Engage your pelvic floor; suck in your navel and subnavel. Use the strength of the inner body to roll slightly forward on your sitting bones. Lift your spine up and out of the pelvic bowl, and allow the natural curvature of your lumbar spine to be expressed. Tuck your chin down, and elevate your sternum toward your chin. Widen your shoulders and press downward with your hands, lengthening the space between your shoulder blades. Draw your thighbones into their sockets, and roll your thighs toward each other to facilitate a hint of internal rotation. Align the bases of your big toes and flex your feet. Stay here for five breaths.

Dandasana is the root of all seated poses, so align your body as close to a neutral point as possible. Feel the inner alignment as well as the outer form.

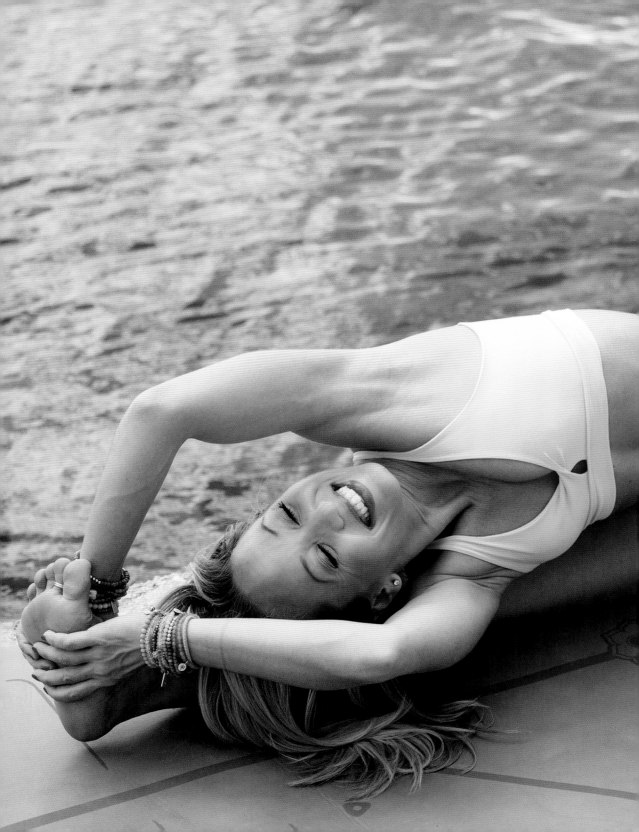

Breaking the Samskara Chain

Students would frequently ask Shri K. Pattabhi Jois about general tightness and inflexibility in the body, and he would often respond with a perplexing statement. Rather than addressing the body, Guruji would simply say, "Oh many samskaras are there," and move on. This left the students wondering where and what these "samskaras" were and why they had so many of them. What Guruji meant is that the students had many past experiences or traumas stored in their bodies and minds, and this psychospiritual patterning was the source of their physical stiffness when practicing yoga. With a little exploration into the Yoga Sutras, it is easy to find that the concept of the samskaras is essential to yoga philosophy. It is also easy to see that we all have many of these samskaras, just like Guruji said!

Every moment, we have the opportunity of experiencing life with a fresh view, but very often we live our lives according to habits and patterns established in the past. Once these patterns are imprinted in our consciousness, they can be very stubborn and tough to change. The Sanskrit word for these repetitive patterns is *samskara*. Samskaras run on autopilot and unconsciously generate the same cyclical type of interactions in the world.

Actions that we take based on past experiences fuel a vicious cycle that builds powerful momentum and forces the cycle to repeat indefinitely. This series of actions and reactions is sometimes known as the "wheel of karma." Whenever you have a deeply ingrained, habitual response to an event, it generates a proclivity for accumulating more of that same type of experience in the present and future. While consciously you may state a desire to be free from a destructive pattern of action and reaction, the patterning is often so deeply rooted in your subconscious mind that it happens without you ever really being aware of it. A common analogy defining negative samskaras likens them to almonds planted in the field of consciousness; when given the fertile ground of attachment and aversion, they ultimately bear the fruit of suffering.

A person can accumulate positive and negative samskaras, and the choice you make about what thoughts, emotions, and actions you take will determine whether your life will be peaceful or painful. Three things are useful for understanding how to work with samskaras. First, just when you think you are in the clear of some old stuff from the past, it comes at you like an undertow. Second, the more you fight it, the worse it gets. Third, all of your habitual responses to fight for or against it will only pull you deeper. This feature can usually be seen as a relapse or a kind of slippery recidivism that pulls you down just when you think you are past a particular issue. So much of your life is driven by subconscious behavioral patterns that it can feel like you are tiptoeing through an emotional minefield.

Yoga seeks to reveal even the sleeping samskaras hidden deep within the body. In contrast to the approach taken by psychotherapy, yoga never demands to know why or where the samskaras come from—you just need to experience them and bring them up into the light of knowledge. If you think you are special and do not have any samskaras, just wait; there is a yoga pose or life experience that will push you to your edge. Then your yoga training actually begins. Take the first step along the inner journey of yoga and see your own samskaras. When you meet them, do not fight them—just experience them, see them, and look at them with compassion and love. Remain with equanimity, observe with an objective mind and an open heart. Once you see a pattern clearly, you want to make amends for the suffering that you have generated through that samskara.

The fire of purification in the practice of yoga is also ultimately the light of clarity. Once you come out of your denial and see the negative samskara's effect on your life, your heart breaks. The tender, achy quality of your heart opens in that moment of realization because you see clearly how your actions have harmed those you love, and you feel empathy for their pain. The power of yoga will burn off the negative samskaras with grace and clarity, and as each samskara is purified, you will walk down the path of life with a little less weight on your back.

1. Examine your personality. What aspect of your personality feeds your samskaras? Identifying key habitual patterns based on past traumas, hurt, or life experiences is a crucial step in the self-awareness needed to burn up the samskaras. You may find yourself comfortable in one of the roles of victim, rescuer, or perpetrator. Look at any rants or diatribes that you have gone on recently to help you identify your samskaras.

2. Press pause. Learning how to walk away from a situation that has a powerful pull on you is sometimes an important lesson in working with the samskaras. If each time you feel the tug to lash out in aggression, fall into depression, or give in to anxiety you pause long enough to break the cycle, you will be making dramatic headway toward addressing the samskaras. Simply not feeding the fire or winding yourself up again will help you defuse the inertia that accumulates when you act out your negative patterns.

3. Plant new seeds. Develop new samskaras that are stronger than the old ones. Replace old habits with new ones that are less harmful. For example, if you have an anger problem and frequently lose your temper, then instead of blowing up at the first trigger, you might try to develop a new samskara by which you take ten deep breaths before any action.

1. *Parighasana*—Gate Pose

Parighasana is an intense side stretch that requires a deep flexion of the hip joints. Named for the iron bar that holds a gate shut, the symbol of a gate on the spiritual path can signify crossing a boundary, entering new territory, or descending to inner chambers. Conversely, it can also symbolize closing doors or leaving old habits and patterns behind. The effort in yoga is often concentrated on removing and burning old samskaras, closing old gates, and opening to new possibilities.

Start in Dandasana. Fold your left leg back and align your left knee forward in line with your left hip joint. Rotate your hips inward and point your left foot back. Open your right leg out to the side at a ninety-degree angle from your left leg. Inhale as you place your hands on your hips to prepare. Suck in your lower belly, engage your pelvic floor, and create space between your ribs and hips. Exhale as you fold your torso forward between your thighs by flexing your hips deeply. Twist your torso back around your right thigh and pull your right lower ribs forward. Spiral your torso around the center line and reach your hands toward your right foot. Interlace your fingers around the sole of your foot and lift your right elbow off the ground. If you cannot hold your foot, then simply lean over to the right as much as possible. Avoid hiking your left hip to go deeper; keep your left hip grounded with a strong awareness of the inner space of your pelvis. Gaze up toward the toes of your right foot to fully enter Parighasana. Stay here for five breaths.

Inhale as you come up, returning your hands to your waist. Exhale and settle into your pelvic floor. Take your hands to the ground, inhale and lift up, and exhale as you jump back to Chaturanga Dandasana. Inhale and come forward to Urdhva Mukha Svanasana; exhale and roll back to Adho Mukha Svanasana. Jump through and repeat the pose on the opposite side.

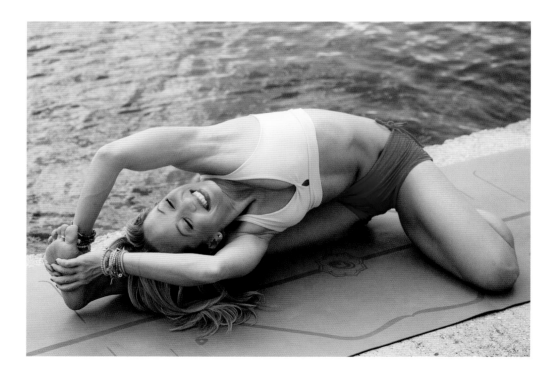

2. *Ardha Matsyendrasana*—Half Lord of the Fishes Pose

Ardha Matsyendrasana is named after the sage Matsyendranath, who is credited as the founder of the Hatha Yoga tradition and is one of the eighty-four *mahasiddhas*. Matsyendranath burned up many of his own samskaras through intensive yoga practice. Doing this deep twist implies a balance between the earthly and the divine.

Start in Dandasana. Fold your right leg under the left and step the left foot over. Align your left foot on the ground close to your right knee, and stand the left leg up. Point your right foot and place it on the ground just to the outside of your right hip. Inhale and make space behind your subnavel; exhale as you fold your body around your left thigh. Drop your right shoulder and rotate the shoulder joint inward. Reach your left arm around your back toward upper right thigh, or as far around toward the right as possible. Ground your hips and look over your left shoulder to fully enter Ardha Matsyendrasana. Come back to Dandasana and repeat on the other side.

Rather than just twisting to the side, think about twisting into your center by using both the core strength of your body and the flexibility of your spine and torso. This pose requires a deep rotation of your hips as well as your shoulders, and you will need the support of the inner body to fully stabilize Ardha Matsyendrasana and balance strength with flexibility.

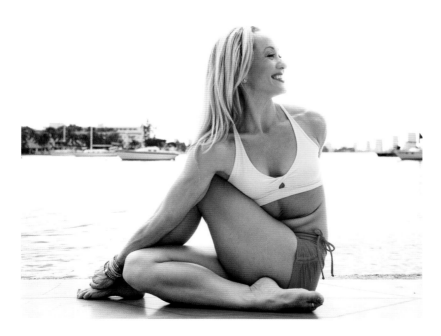

In the Ashtanga Yoga tradition, this posture in the Intermediate Series is used to reestablish your connection to your core and literally twist into your center after the deep backbends of the Ashtanga Yoga Second Series. This twist can also be used to facilitate internal rotation of the hips, relieve shoulder stress, and encourage healthy digestion.

3. *Ubhaya Padangusthasana*—Double Big Toe Pose

The traditional entry into Ubhaya Padangusthasana requires that you roll up through your spine, like a gently rolling wheel. *Ubhaya* means "both," and you maintain a firm grip on both big toes throughout the pose. The samskara cycle is often represented as a giant wheel turning and gaining momentum without any conscious awareness or control. By learning to roll through the spine, yogis at least gain control of their own bodies and, hopefully, one day lessen the inertia of old samskaras.

Start in Dandasana. Exhale and roll back to a supine position. Inhale and take your legs over your head as in Halasana. Wrap your index and middle fingers and your thumbs around your big toes. Exhale here while rolling slightly back onto the balls of your feet. Inhale and roll up to Ubhaya Padangusthasana. Straighten the arms and leg, gaze upward, and allow your head to tilt slightly back to facilitate the gaze. While rolling through your spine, do not pull with your arms. Instead suck in your belly, draw in your ribs, and use the strength in the center of your pelvis to control the movement. If you pull with your arms, you will often lose your grip and miss the key steps of inner awareness along the central axis. If you reach a point where you seem to tip backward, ground through your sitting bones and point your toes to bring your weight slightly forward. Stay here for five breaths.

If after three rolls you do not make it up to the full pose, then release your feet, sit up, and enter Ubhaya Padangusthasana from a seated position. From Dandasana bend your knees and lean slightly back to lift your legs. Grab hold of your big toes and slowly straighten your legs by drawing the thighbones into their sockets. Stay here for five breaths.

Exhale and return to Dandasana, cross your feet, and jump back to Chaturanga Dandasana. Inhale as you come forward to Urdhva Mukha Svanasana, then exhale and roll back to Adho Mukha Svanasana.

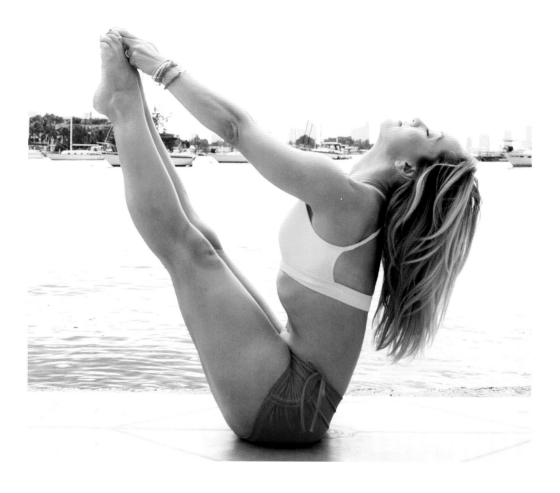

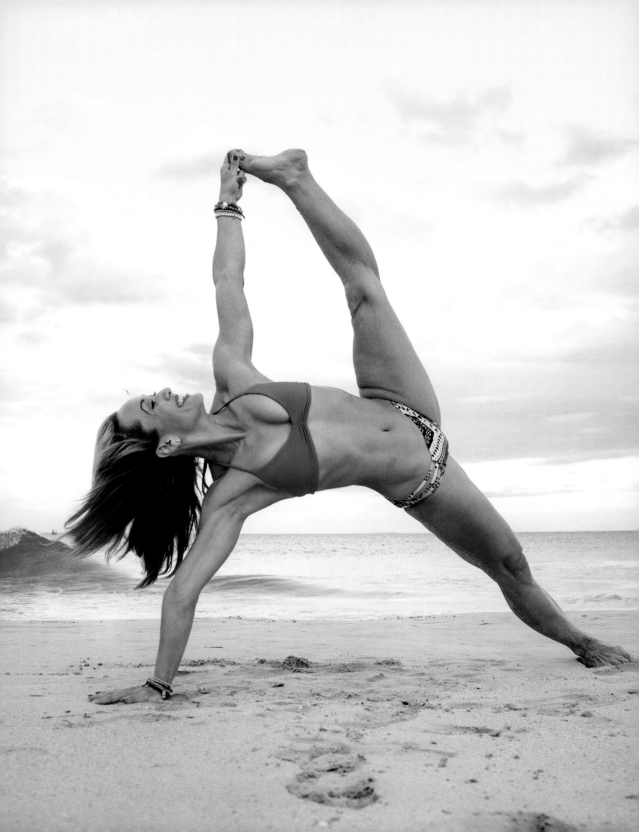

Being Happy
Saumanasya

The health of a tree is shown in the sweetness of its fruits. Similarly, the efficacy of the yoga path is embodied by the yogi's cheerful disposition. This state of happiness is the mark of a lifelong commitment to the spiritual path—and it is today's yogi assignment.

Known in Sanskrit as *saumanasya*, the yogic state of happiness is a cheerful contentment and pleasant attitude toward life. You can spend your whole life searching outside yourself for happiness, but if you find it inside yourself, you will then illuminate the world with the brightness of your light. Patanjali's Yoga Sutras outline the evidence of a lifelong commitment to yoga. Yoga Sutra 2.41 states that the yogi's mind rests in pure and peaceful subtle awareness (*sattva*), has been purified (*suddhi*), maintains a cheerful attitude (*saumanasya*), concentrates on a single point of attention (*ekagra*), has mastery over the five senses (*indriya jaya*), and is able to directly experience the true self (*atma-darshan*). These are the fruits of the yoga path. Far more important that any physical pose, it is this orientation toward the innermost truth that produces lasting happiness.

Taking the time to get on your mat and practice is sometimes the first step in creating the yogi's cheerful attitude. If you find yourself caught in a cycle of negativity and are unable to see the positive, it is often because you have not made time for yourself to heal, nourish, or process. It can be hard to take time out for yourself when you are consumed by the busyness of life, so when your body sends you a distress signal, it can be easier to ignore it than to listen. Carving out time for practice, even just five minutes, is a statement of self-worth, a statement that says, "I am worth these five minutes of self-care."

It's easy to complain about the infinite number of annoying things that can happen at any given time during any given day, but if you let yourself get sucked into that mind-set, you will miss the magic of life. Spending the precious moments of your life in misery is a waste.

You have a choice about how you think, feel, and live. Emotions are practiced and patterned; you can build a habit pattern of complaint or you can build a habit pattern of cheerfulness. If you are stuck in a traffic jam, instead of wallowing in your misery, take the opportunity to appreciate your car, the person you are with, or the city you live in. If you are dealing with a difficult family situation, take the time to remember how much you love your family and how much they add to your life. Smile from your heart at least once a day. Let the good cheer from your heart spill out into your whole life—let it change your world.

Your happiness depends on you. Take responsibility for your inner state of being and decide to get really, really happy. Sing your heart's joy like a full-on symphonic overture. Smile so brightly that the people around cannot help but smile with you.

HOMEWORK

1. Define your view of happiness. Reflect on what happiness means for you. Define it in your own terms, not anyone else's. Maybe happiness is your yoga practice, maybe it's the beach, maybe it's building custom motorcycles, maybe it's going to law school, maybe it's being a parent. Or maybe happiness is finally being comfortable in your own skin.

2. Share happiness. Smile at someone you don't know today, give someone a hug, pay someone a compliment. Laugh, love, be happy.

3. Listen. Notice how many times a day you complain, curse, or shake your head at others, yourself, or your world. Stop yourself before you engage in a negative attitude and see if there is something deeper bothering you. Look at the underlying issues that stand between you and a state of saumanasya. Maybe that means making time to seek treatment for an ailment that you have been ignoring or setting some boundaries to claim personal space or more free time for yourself. If you feel overextended because you have taken on too much, or if you are feeling taken advantage of, then self-care can mean taking time back for yourself. If there are things you need to get done that you have been avoiding, knocking those things off your to-do list will lift a huge burden from you.

1. *Uttana Shishosana*—Extended Puppy Pose

This relatively simple pose is a wonderful way to tune in to the playful, happy spirit of youth. Instead of the Downward-Facing Dog, this is the Puppy. Like a puppy, you are meant to have a cheerful heart while exploring the inner body.

Start off on your hands and knees. Walk your hands forward, looking toward your fingertips, and allow your chest to descend to the ground. If your shoulders are tight, tuck your head and reach your forehead to the ground. Allow your chin to rest comfortably on the ground, and open your armpits downward. Suck your navel back into the emptiness of your pelvis and allow your spine to drape down, out of your pelvic bowl. Stay here for five breaths, then lean back and rest in Balasana. Repeat up to three times.

Uttana Shishosana can help relieve lower back pain and release the spine, especially for people who have tight hamstrings and cannot successfully access Adho Mukha Svanasana.

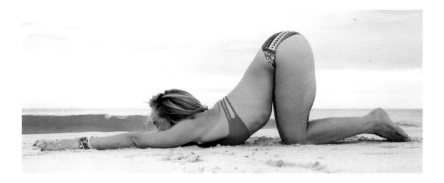

2. *Bharadvajasana*—Pose Dedicated to the Sage Bharadvaja

Named after the historic sage Bharadvaja, this twist offers yogis a chance to cultivate a peaceful mind. Bharadvaja is considered one of the seven seers of our modern era. He lived during the Vedic times, excelled at scholarship, and attained deep states of meditation. He is often depicted with one leg folded into Half Lotus and the other leg hidden behind him, and the foundation of this twisting pose is based on this traditional representation. When practicing Bharadvajasana, align yourself with your deeper spiritual journey toward knowledge and higher consciousness.

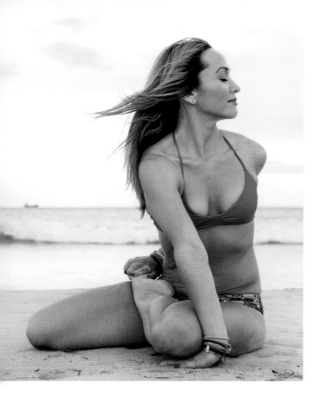

Start in Dandasana. Fold your right leg back by rotating your right hip joint inward. Align your right foot with the outer edge of your right hip and point your toes. Open your right leg at a forty-five-degree angle from your public bone, and settle your hips toward the ground. Fold your left leg into Half Lotus by rotating it outward, and place the instep of your left foot along your right hip crease. If you cannot fold your leg into Half Lotus, simply bend your left knee and drape your left foot close to your right knee. Open your left leg out to the left side at a forty-five-degree angle from your pubic bone. Inhale and suck in your navel and subnavel; maximize the space between your ribs and hips. Exhale as you twist to the left. Reach your left hand toward your left foot, clasping it as firmly as possible. Place your right hand under your left knee, aligning the heel of your hand with the outer edge of your thigh; press down firmly. Roll your right shoulder inward and your left shoulder outward; gaze over your left shoulder. Stay here for five breaths.

Inhale as you return to Dandasana, and cross your feet to lift up. Exhale and jump back to Chaturanga Dandasana. Inhale as you come forward to Urdhva Mukha Svanasana; exhale as you roll back to Adho Mukha Svanasana. Jump through and repeat the pose on the opposite side.

3. *Vashisthasana*—Side Plank Pose

Named after the great sage Vashistha, this side arm balance helps you find the center line and keep the mind focused on the true source of happiness within. Vashistha was one of the seven great *rishis*, according to traditional Vedic philosophy. He is credited with being happily married to Arundhati and made content with the possession of the divine cow Nandini, which was able to grant his every wish and provide for him indefinitely. Vashistha refused to trade Nandini to the sage Visvamitra (who was King Kaushika at the time) for all the riches of the world, leading to a legendary feud between the two sages. It could be argued that Vashistha resisted the temptation of worldly riches in favor of his sacred cow, the embodiment of his relationship with God, who provides all things. For practitioners of yoga, a similar shift in perspective eventually happens as the heart and mind discover the true source of sustenance within.

Start in Utthita Chaturanga Dandasana. Roll to the right to make a side version of the pose. Shift your right hand slightly forward, about one hand-length in front of your right shoulder. Align your right hand and right foot. Come up onto the outer edge of your right foot. Stack your body along the center line by drawing in your ribs and engaging your lower abdominal muscles. At first, find your balance by keeping your left arm tucked into the left side of your body. Once you can maintain your balance, extend your left arm upward, keeping your shoulders in line with each other. Gaze toward the fingertips of your left hand. Once you attain balance again, lift your left leg through by rotating the left hip joint outward. Do not lift your left leg merely by opening your inner thighs. Your left hip joint must roll outward to facilitate the maximum lift of your leg. As your left hip spirals out to the side, the head of the thighbone drops deeper into the socket, and your left foot reaches up close to your left hand. If possible, wrap your first three fingers around your left big toe and bind the pose to fully enter

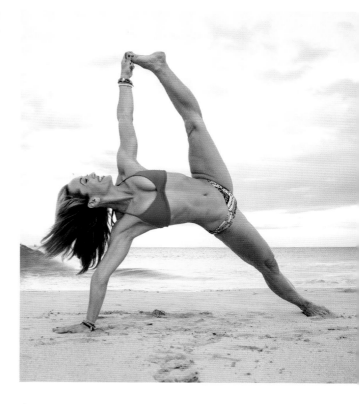

Vashisthasana. Stay here for five breaths, gazing up toward your left hand. Feel welcome to stop at any stage along the way based on your level of strength and flexibility.

Exhale as you lower your left leg. Inhale to stabilize your pelvic floor. Exhale as you lower your left arm back to its original side position and then turn and put your hand all the way back down to the ground in Utthita Chaturanga Dandasana. Inhale and roll forward immediately to Urdhva Mukha Svanasana; exhale and roll back to Adho Mukha Svanasana. Come forward to Utthita Chaturanga Dandasana again and repeat Vashisthasana on the left side.

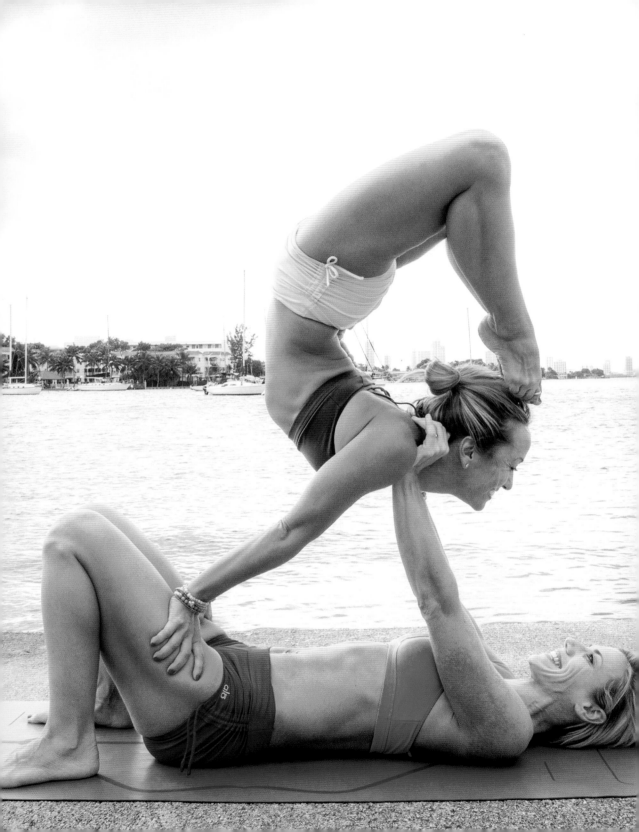

Yoga Friends
Sangha

My life before yoga consisted of all-night parties, dance music, and generally being too fabulous for my own good. I had a lot of high heels and makeup paired with plenty of attitude and ego. I never thought I would give all that up for early-morning yoga practice. A life-changing moment happened one day when I was in an elevator going to an after-hours party on an average Monday morning. A man in his midfifties was reminiscing about the party scene of the 1980s, which was filled with cocaine and heroin. It hit me like an epiphany that endless raves would only lead me to be like him. I would either be in my midfifties holding on to the almost glorious party days of the ecstasy generation, or I would have to do something "real" with my life.

It was another year before I took any significant action, but I slowly started to see that my hunger for sleepless nights spent on the dance floor, fueled by chemical substances, was a kind of spiritual desperation. I had been struggling with my own sadness since I was nine years old. I was miserable, and I never had the tools to face my own misery. When I first took ecstasy, it was like a kind of happiness that I had never felt in my life. So I did more and more of it in a mad dash to self-medicate the then-undiagnosed depression from which I had been suffering for most of my life. There are many problems with self-medicating a psychiatric disorder using a controlled illegal substance, starting with the most obvious that reliance on drugs creates an addictive cycle that can wreck your whole life. On the quest for a bigger high, I was on the road to self-destruction. It was an endless train that I may not have gotten off if I had not met that man in the elevator. I guess that in some ways I owe him a debt of gratitude.

The seed of change was planted in my heart. I wanted to live a more peaceful life. I wanted to be genuinely nice and let go of my self-importance and sense of entitlement. I made a series of decisions to get my life back on track. But it all began with the decision that I was worth it, that my life was worth saving, and that I had value as a human being. I took the GREs, applied to graduate school at New York University, and joined an Ashtanga Yoga class. I was overwhelmed during my first yoga class. Not only was everyone nice, but I felt something completely new. Lying in the final relaxation at the end of class, I felt comfortable in my own skin. The discomfort I had known my whole life, like a discordant tune of angst playing in the background of every situation I had ever experienced, was finally gone. I knew that this was the real "high."

The first casualties of my new lifestyle were my party friends. While I knew that this new path was the right one for me, I felt like I was walking a solitary journey. Within a few months of that first yoga class, I moved to New York City and joined a traditional Ashtanga Yoga Mysore Style class. The teacher told me to come six days a week at eight in the morning. My world literally turned on its axis; 8:00 A.M. was when I used to arrive at the best, most exclusive after-parties! Committing myself to yoga meant changing my life in ways that I wanted but was not truly prepared for. Not only did I move away from Miami and immerse myself in an intensive graduate studies program, but suddenly I was going to bed before midnight and doing yoga at what felt like the crack of dawn. If it were not for the welcoming community of Ashtangis in New York, I do not think I would have been able to stick with the spiritual path. I needed a *sangha*, a spiritual community to guide my transition to the yoga life.

When I finished my first practice in New York, there were women in the changing room who invited me out for juice. When I didn't show up on a Sunday for practice because some party friends visited me in New York, everyone noticed I was not there. When I saw that all the yogis drank green juices and brought healthy snacks, I questioned my diet. When two students from my class went to India to study with Shri K. Pattabhi Jois, I asked my teacher about it, and he encouraged me to read Guruji's book and go to India. My life changed; not only did I find my sangha, but I found my life's path. Without the genuine support of the yoga community, I would not have made it.

Today's yogi assignment is sangha, the spiritual community or yoga friends. It is so important to have friends who understand and support your practice, who will applaud you for getting up at 5:00 A.M. and dragging yourself to practice. Yoga friends are happy to celebrate and lift their glasses to cheer with green juice and a handstand instead of wine and cigarettes. You need someone to commiserate with about your failed headstand and to celebrate your first backbend. It can be hard for people who do not practice to understand why you are nearly in tears just because you balanced on your head for a few seconds today.

But the yoga community is not heaven, so don't come to it looking for angels. The yoga world is made up of human beings. I do not want to paint a rosy view of a world that still has gossip, scandal, power, fame, and money in it. Yogis, however, are held to a higher standard. As a yoga practitioner, you must ask yourself what it means to live the yoga life. More than anything, yoga is a commitment to live a peaceful life and to change your world. It takes strength, steadiness, and determination.

The spiritual path is not a competition where fellow yogis duke it out for the top spot. It is a journey on which we reach out and lift each other up. We are not here to glorify ourselves but to chip away at the chains of ego, pride, and jealousy. We are here to be humble, to be kind, to learn how to take the higher road, to drop the fighting and forcing, and to end the emotional warfare that only engenders more conflict. There is no uniform, no particular outfit, no size, shape, age, gender, ethnicity, or social class that makes you a yogi. It is what is in your heart. When you are in alignment, your heart sings with joy. When you take action that is out of alignment, your heart registers this lack of integrity. As a yogi, when you feel this irresolution, take action to right the wrong. Be a good yoga friend.

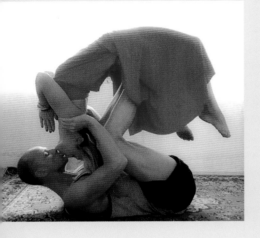

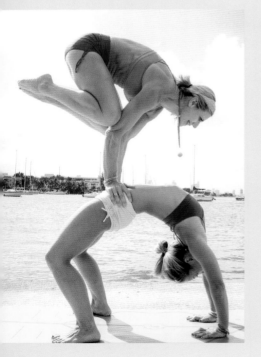

1. Identify your yoga friends. Reach out to them today and invite them to share a practice, a juice, or a vegan meal. Practice together, join an acro-yoga class, or help each other with partner work to build a sense of shared trust.

I dedicate this assignment to my two best yoga friends. The first is my husband, Tim. Throughout our marriage, we have shared multiple trips to India, the heart and spirit of the practice, and we opened a yoga center together in Miami. We share love and life. The second is Kerri Verna, whom many people know as @beachyogagirl on Instagram. Truly, she's my best friend, and I would not be able to walk this path without her. Who are your yoga friends?

2. Find your yoga values. Identify three core values that you think define the yoga sangha. For example, they could be peace, strength, and authenticity. Then open the dialogue with your community of yoga friends and find out what shared values you embrace.

3. Be a yoga friend. Next time you go to class, look for the newbies and welcome them into the community by inviting them for a juice or just letting them know that you are there for them. Or find people online who are new to the practice. Follow their accounts on Instagram, and offer kind words of encouragement while letting them know that they have a friend on the yoga path.

4. Form a virtual sangha. Join a social media group that shares your values. Share your story honestly and provide sustenance for the journey through friendship and support.

1. Join a yoga sangha.

Go to class! I have not given you a series of poses for today's practice. Instead, I want you to go to an actual, physical class and meet a local teacher and community of yogis.

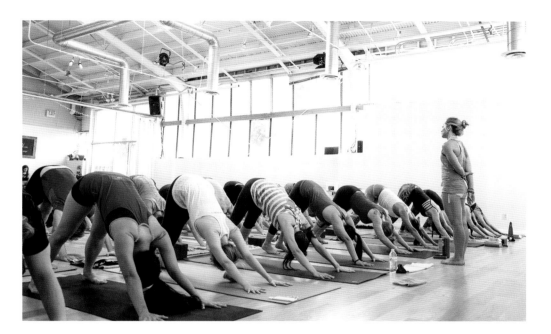

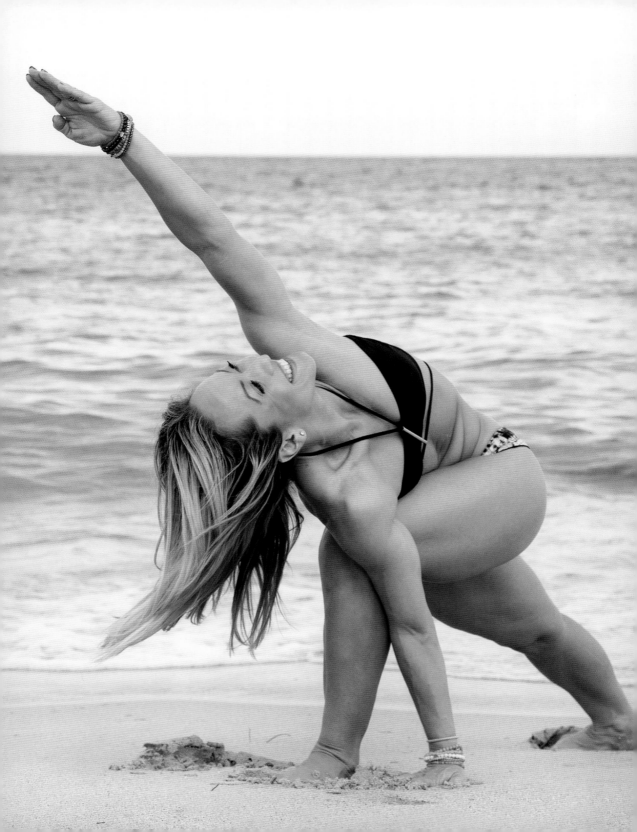

Memory
Smrti

always hated rote memorization in school. My distaste for memorization was actually one of the reasons that I chose to study literature. I nearly flunked an Advanced Placement biology test because I simply could not make myself sit down and memorize the bones and muscles of the human body. There are two ironies here. First, thanks to nearly twenty years of yoga practice and teaching, I now have most of those bones and muscles memorized. My high school biology teacher would be proud! And second, not to toot my own horn, but I actually have a really good memory. I retain what I read with above-average detail as long as I pay attention while I'm reading. My brain acts as a repository for random facts accumulated through years of education, reading, and general studying. I would actually like to erase some of those files, but it turns out that memory is not selective like a computer hard drive. Perhaps it is fitting that the most traditional way of practicing Ashtanga Yoga asks the student to memorize the order of the poses.

Ashtanga Yoga has a reputation for being dogmatic and demanding—and it certainly is demanding. But whether it is dogmatic really depends on who is teaching. You may wonder how you can be demanding without being dogmatic. Ashtanga Yoga requires that students who practice the traditional Mysore Style method memorize the order of the poses. Students are often allowed a cheat sheet for a few days, but some teachers will not even permit that. Then students are asked to maintain a six-day-a-week practice. If you want to progress to the more advanced poses, there is no gray zone about whether or not you have to meet these two requirements. Usually students balk at the idea of memorizing a sequence. They either rebel against the idea of doing the same thing every day, or they fear the need to commit the poses to memory. Repetition is really the key to success. Most Olympic athletes have their training program memorized, repeat the same moves over and over, and follow their coaches' guidance.

The role of memory in traditional yoga studies cannot be overestimated. The entire teaching of the Yoga Sutras first began as an oral tradition that was committed to memory through the vehicle of chanting for nearly five hundred years before it was secured in written form. The ability of the yoga aspirant to commit large chunks of knowledge to memory was considered to be a test of discipline and fortitude. Retaining 196 aphorisms spanning four books was a necessary requirement for all would-be students of yoga in the most historical sense. Prior to any inquiry about the reason or logic of yoga's most fundamental philosophical text, practitioners were required to memorize the entire volume of Patanjali's work. Imagine if contemporary teachers demanded the same from their students today! The ranks of yoga students would certainly dwindle.

Memorizing the poses shifts your attention to the inner body. By committing the series to memory, you create the space for your mind to draw its full attention inward. As long as you are focused outside yourself, following a teacher for instructions and wondering what comes next, the mind will always be turned slightly outward. Once the poses are memorized, your mind can focus entirely within. Plus the series of poses assimilates into the subconscious mind where deeper learning takes place.

Memory is so fungible and our desire for personal protection so strong that we can actually block out whole experiences from our awareness. How you engage with memory is how you engage with your mind and body, and the two together are the vehicle for the journey of yoga. No matter what your life experience actually is, what you take away from the events that you live through is a larger factor in determining your personal state of happiness. I have a tendency to skew toward the negative, to remember the arguments rather than the good times. Through yoga, I have learned to train my perception to be more neutral, objective, and truthful.

Today's yogi assignment is memory (*smrti*). Three types of memory play a big role in the spiritual path. First, you can remember the words of your teacher in moments of distress along the yoga path. Second, you can remember the sacred teaching of the primary texts of your spiritual lineage, which are your armor in difficult situations. Finally, and most important, you will ultimately remember your true self. Yoga philosophy says that each of us carries an eternal self within and that no matter how deeply it is buried under the mountain of personal doubt, there is a memory of that true self. Through the practice, the light of your true self begins to shine through, and you wake up to the memory of who you really are.

1. Remember the words of your teacher. Write down a key phrase that you have heard your teacher say. Tape it up on your desk, or take a screenshot and store it on your phone where you will see it often. Use this memory to inspire your practice.

2. Keep your perspective. Remember how far you have come along the path! Take time to reflect on a key turning point in your life, whether it was deciding to practice yoga, meeting your life partner, choosing your job or school, or some other important event in your life. Be as objective as possible, and notice any tendency to view the event in an overly positive or overly negative way. Note the steps you have taken forward since that key turning point.

3. Practice memorization. Commit one of the Yoga Sutras to memory. Start off with the translation in your native language, and then memorize the sutra in its original Sanskrit. Add one new sutra per week as your goal until you reach the completion of Book One of the Yoga Sutras.

HOMEWORK

1. *Parivrtta Parsvakonasana*—Revolved Extended Side-Angle Pose
This standing pose is rather challenging. Not only is a high degree of flexibility required, but the mind must maintain multiple points of awareness, most of which remain out of sight while you complete the full pose.

Start in Samasthiti. Spread your legs relatively wide, keeping a distance of about one leg-length between your feet. This distance is adjustable based on your height, leg length, and level of flexibility. Align your left heel with your right arch, and turn your hips to the left. If possible, keep your right heel planted. If that is not possible, then completely square your hips and come forward onto the ball of your right foot. The balance may be more precarious, and if you feel yourself teetering, sink your right knee to the ground for greater stability.

Your legs provide the foundation for this pose, and you have three options to choose from based on your level of flexibility and balance. As you enter the pose, be diligent in remembering your foundation. Keep a

PRACTICE

MEMORY SMRTI

sense of grounding through your right leg and reach all the way down through either the ball or the outer edge of the foot, depending on which option suits your practice. Keep your pelvic floor constantly activated. Choosing one of the three foundations, prepare to enter Parivrtta Parsvakonasana B by drawing in your navel and subnavel and lean toward the left on an inhalation. Exhale as you fold your torso completely around your left thigh. Deepen the left hip crease and encourage a comfortable hip flexion on the left side. Allow your left hip joint to spiral in a gentle internal rotation. Fold your chest, ribs, and shoulders all the way around your left thigh. Plant your right hand on the ground and point the fingers in the same direction as the toes on your left foot to fully enter Parivrtta Parsvakonasana B. If you cannot reach the ground, place a block along the outer edge of your left foot and rest your hand on that. Your right shoulder folds inward while your left shoulder extends upward and rolls outward. Gaze at the fingers of your left hand. Your entire body will remain out of sight, so you have to use internal feeling and memory to hold the alignment steady. Stay here for five breaths. Inhale as you come up and immediately repeat on the other side. Stay here for five breaths, then inhale, come up, and return to Samasthiti.

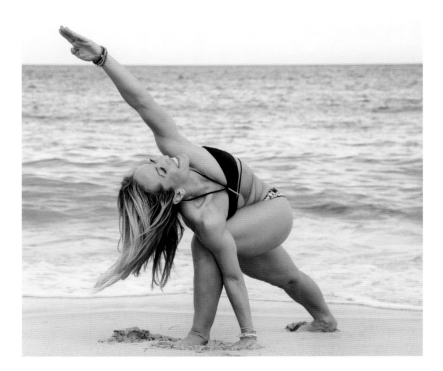

2. *Purvottanasana*—Upward Plank Pose

Purvottanasana translates directly into English as "intense east stretch." It pairs with Paschimattanasana, which literally means "intense west stretch."

Start in Dandasana. Exhale as you suck in your lower belly, tuck your tailbone, and round your lower back. Point your toes, activate your quadriceps, and rotate your hips inward. Walk your hands back about six inches from your hips. Point your fingers toward your toes and rotate your shoulders inward. Now lift your chest and tuck your chin into your sternum. Inhale as you engage your pelvic floor and send your hips powerfully up and forward. Maintain a healthy activation of your quadriceps. As your hips lift, your feet naturally come down to the floor, but do not try to touch them to the floor or you may get a cramp in your calves or toes. Keep your chin tucked into your chest for a brief moment to check your subnavel. Pooching the lower belly is a common misalignment that happens in Purvottanasana; it can easily be corrected by keeping a conscious awareness of the area. When you feel confident in your lower belly's ability to stay drawn into the inner space of your pelvis, drop your head back and gaze toward your nose. Keeping your shoulders rolled inward creates a natural support for your neck by elevating your trapezius muscles. Maintain a conscious awareness of your whole body to remember the key alignment points. Even though you cannot see your body, keep it firmly in your mind. Stay here for five breaths, then return to Dandasana.

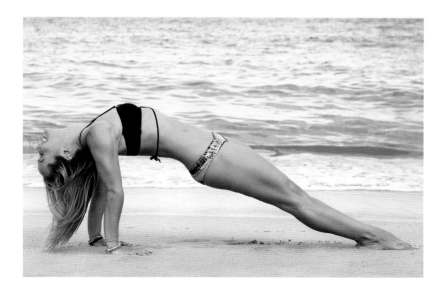

3. *Baddha Padmasana*—Bound Lotus Pose

Baddha means "bind," and another way to think of memory is binding an image or idea in your mind. Baddha Padmasana is traditionally used as part of the Closing Poses of the Ashtanga Yoga tradition. It is usually meant to signify the binding or locking in of the intensive inner work of the practice. The lotus (*padma*) is a symbol of spiritual growth and awakening. One of the most commonly experienced obstacles along the yoga path is recidivism. Binding the lotus at the end of the practice is an effort at maintaining whatever ground has been gained along the inner path.

Start in Dandasana. Fold your legs into a comfortable seated pose. If you cannot sit cross-legged comfortably, then do not proceed to the full pose. Instead, wrap your arms around your back and hold your elbows. If you can sit comfortably in a cross-legged pose, you may be able to fold your legs into Padmasana. Start by folding your right leg into Half Lotus. Aim the instep of your right foot toward your left hip crease. Check in with your right knee and be sure it feels good before proceeding. If not, remove your right foot from the pose. If you are ready to move on, fold your left foot into Half Lotus and aim the instep

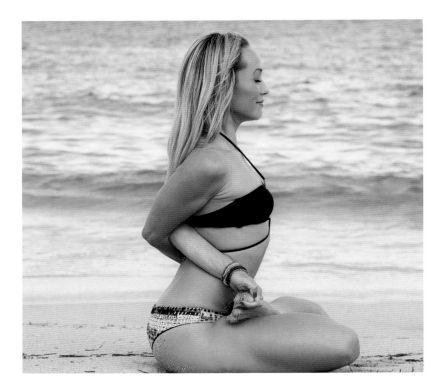

toward your right hip crease. Lift your left foot over your right shin but keep your left knee joint closed as you enter Padmasana. Be sure your heels remain on the inside of the iliac crests. Avoid sickling your feet (as in dance, with toes pointing inward and heels outward) or allowing them to slide down toward the floor. Activate your feet slightly, but do not flex them. If you are comfortable in Padmasana, then proceed to bind your lotus. Reach around your back with your left arm and aim the hand toward the top of your left foot. If you cannot reach your foot, simply leave your hand in the air reaching as far toward your foot as you can. Reach you right arm around your back on top of your left arm and aim your right hand toward the top of your right foot. When you bind both of your feet, you have entered full Baddha Padmasana.

To deepen the pose, you can lock your elbows on top of each other and create an even tighter bind. However, this is only recommended for very flexible students or students of the Ashtanga Yoga Intermediate Series. Stay here for ten breaths, then either inhale and release or move immediately into the traditional Closing Poses (as outlined in both volumes of *The Power of Ashtanga Yoga*).

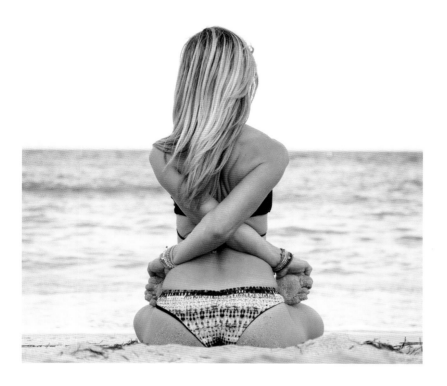

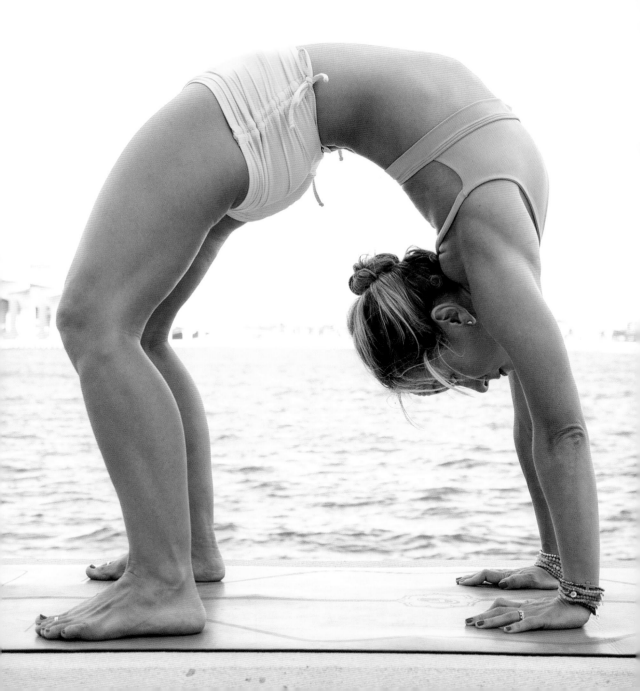

The Acceptance of Pain
Tapas

here is a pain I feel when my alarm goes off at 5:00 A.M.; I accept it. There is a pain I feel burning in my abs when I hold Chaturanga Dandasana for longer than usual; I accept it. There is a pain I feel when, because of an injury, I have to modify my practice and take it easy; I accept it. I do not run away from these types of pain.

People ask me all the time how I got so flexible and strong. The simple and easy answer is that I have been practicing every day for nearly twenty years. I was not naturally good at yoga; I couldn't touch my toes, bend my back, or do a headstand when I started. But through devotion, dedication, and determination, I have experienced a slow, steady shift from the impossible to the possible. In traditional yoga philosophy, this is called *tapas*, literally translated as "heat," which means the discipline to accept the necessary suffering encountered along the yoga path. Practicing yoga is like submitting yourself to the fire of purification.

Today's yogi assignment is tapas. Sometimes defined as asceticism or discipline, another way to think of tapas is the acceptance of pain that leads to purification. Physical, mental, and spiritual tapas builds the strength and determination that give you the power to achieve your life goals. Success is as much a result of hard work as it is of talent and luck. You already have everything you need in your heart to succeed in yoga and in life. Through the power of tapas, you learn to access your natural power and truly be strong. Tapas can be making the commitment to do something that is difficult for you in service of the practice, like getting up early or doing a posture that you always avoid. Or tapas can be kicking an old habit that is getting in the way of your practice. It can also be the decision to increase the number of days you practice or wake up early (like I did this morning) in service of yoga. In other words, tapas is far more than just physical pain.

According to traditional yoga philosophy, there are a few different types of tapas. First, any activity can be defined according to its categorization within the three *gunas*. The gunas are the fundamental qualities of nature that have always been and will always be present in the world. As such, the yogi can engage in sattvic tapas, rajastic tapas, or tamasic tapas. *Sattvic tapas* is the true yogic state of purification, performed in a calm and equanimous manner with a sustained attitude of nonattachment. *Rajastic tapas* is performed with a fierce intensity and is often associated with ego achievement; it can sometimes lead to unnecessary suffering and will have a mixed effect on the inner state of purification. Finally, *tamasic tapas* is the misconstrued notion of subjecting yourself to extreme states of pain under the guise of purification, even to the extent of torturing or harming yourself. Unfortunately, this does not serve the yogic path and will only further entrench you in a self-directed, punitive cycle of negativity. A good way of discerning under which guna your tapas is performed is to check your intention.

Within the sattvic tapas, there are three more traditional types of tapas: purification of body, speech, and mind. Bodily tapas is maintaining a daily physical discipline that keeps the body as physically pure and energized as possible. This includes following a yogic diet, practicing every day, and caring for and cleaning the body. Tapas of speech means purifying your language and what you choose to say. The yogi speaks only the truth in a kindhearted manner, devoid of all ill-spirited intentions. At the very least, modern-day yogis can edit unnecessary or gratuitous profanity from their speech and refrain from purposely harming another person with insults or hurtful words. Finally, tapas of the mind—which is essentially the yogic effort to maintain a calm and equanimous mind with unbroken attention at a single point in the inner body—is perhaps the greatest effort.

To assist in the practice of all three tapas, R. Sharath Jois often talks about the "four Ds" that you need for correct yoga practice: devotion, dedication, discipline, and determination. It is his way of explaining tapas in action. Yogis have a disciplined life to support the inward direction of the yogic mind. Only with consistent, sustained effort will the real work of yoga happen; that is, old negative thoughts are replaced with positive ones. Sharath says, "If you just keep on doing asanas without thinking about these types of things, then the practice is just like a mindless physical activity with no spiritual use. What is the use of a beautiful physical body if you don't have a good heart or good thinking?" Once you commit to the true spiritual practice and embody the brave heart of a yogi, you will no longer be disturbed by many things in your life. That is the transformation that happens when you do your practice for a long time with dedication and determination. Only with faith and devotion does a practitioner become a *sadhaka*, a yogi who is willing to sacrifice and accept some pain as a necessary part of service on the yoga path.

How we each define pain is simultaneously a semantic discussion and a personal experience. All of us have a different pain threshold and a different level of sensitivity in our bodies, and simply saying that we should never feel pain when we practice disregards the highly personal journey of body awareness. As a general rule during your practice, pain around the joints should be avoided, whereas some muscular sensations of strengthening and stretching that some people may call pain or burning are often physically safe. But even that guideline cannot be universally applied, because not everyone can actually feel their muscles or joints when they practice. One way to think about tapas is to look for the edge of comfortable discomfort, a middle way between harmful physical extremes and excessive caution.

Yoga shines a light deep within the inner space of physical, emotional, and mental bodies and opens a path to healing. We have all experienced firsthand the transformational shifts from the spiritual journey of yoga. It's not always the advanced poses that bring us healing or involve the most powerful tapas. The poses are just windows into the true self, and in the presence of that divine spark, healing happens. The infinite wisdom of true grace is uplifting and humbling, leaving you with faith and surrender as your guiding light, and makes all the tapas totally worth it.

1. Break old habits. Do you have a habit that gets in the way of your practice? Something like smoking, drinking, doing drugs, over- or undereating, getting lost in the online world, or just beating yourself up too much? It will require determination, strength, and the acceptance of pain to change this habit. Commit yourself to making the change today, and willingly submit yourself to the fire of purification. If you have a substance addiction, consider joining a twelve-step recovery program, seeking the guidance of a qualified professional, and asking for help.

2. Practice tapas of speech. Write down each time you curse, swear, or lie throughout the day. Ask yourself if it was truly necessary to do so to communicate your point. Write down each time that you speak in a way that is not aligned with yogic values, such as gossiping, using insults, dredging up the past merely to hurt someone, telling lies, spreading negativity, and so on. Ask yourself why you feel compelled to engage in this mode of conversation, and recognize the underlying hurt you have within that spurs you to communicate in this way.

3. Cultivate new habits. Certain elements of the yoga lifestyle require an element of tapas. Choose one and commit to it for a period of three months. You could choose to practice every day, follow a vegetarian or vegan diet, drink more water, go to bed early, or wake up early.

PRACTICE
1. *Chaturanga Dandasana*—Four-Pointed Staff Pose
This is one of the hardest poses in the Ashtanga Yoga series to practice with good alignment. It is normally held for only one breath throughout the transitions in the practice, because as soon as you attempt to hold it longer, the power of its tapas becomes evident. Guruji and Sharath would often ask their students to hold Chaturanga Dandasana throughout guided Ashtanga Yoga practices as a kind of surprise test of strength and determination. One thing is certain about this pose: your whole body will be dipped into the fire of purification!

Start in Utthita Chaturanga Dandasana, with your feet slightly separated, your weight bearing down through the balls of your feet, your pelvic floor and lower abdominal muscles engaged, your ribs tucked under, and your shoulders spread wide. Slowly exhale as you bend your elbows to lower yourself toward the ground. Allow your body to glide down in the space between your arms while maintaining its strength along the center line. Press continuously with your arms. Allow your chest to sink just below your elbows, and stop bending when your elbows reach ninety-degree angles. Gaze at your nose. Stay here for one breath, then either progress to Urdhva Mukha Svanasana or return to Plank Pose. Repeat this sequence three times.

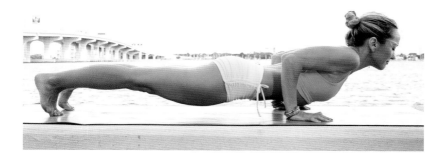

While there is a necessary level of muscular activation in Chaturanga Dandasana, there should be no pain in any of your joints. The tips of your shoulders *must* point forward and not down, or you place undue pressure on the acromion process on your shoulder blades, which can lead to shoulder injuries. Instead, find the support for your shoulder deeper down, in the muscles of the rotator cuff and the power of the latissimus dorsi (back) muscles. If you cannot safely enter Chaturanga Dandasana, then Plank Pose is a healthy and relatively accessible modification.

2. *Urdhva Dhanurasana*—Upward Bow Pose

Often just called a "backbend," Urdhva Dhanurasana is the source of much necessary suffering. Accepting this pose as part of your practice is a kind of tapas.

Start off in a supine position. Bend your knees and elbows. Align your feet just a bit wider than hip-width apart, and place your feet as close to your pelvis as possible. Place your hands under your shoulders, point-ing your fingers toward your toes. Relax the mind. Do not stress doing a full backbend—just taking the time to practice it is enough. Inhale as you send your hips up and forward, and roll onto the top of your head. Pause here for a moment to check your alignment. Track your knees in line with your hips while you send your knees forward on top of your feet. Draw your elbows in so they are in line with your wrists and shoulders. Before you lift into full Urdhva Dhanurasana, pause, breathe, and check the alignment of your torso. Lift your ribs over your head, maximize the space between your ribs and hips, layer your subnavel into your pelvic bowl, and engage your pelvic floor. Inhale as you lift up into Urdhva Dhanurasana. Allow an even distribution of weight between your hips, legs, chest, and arms. Press down with your shoulders equally as you root down with your legs. Stay here for five breaths. Come down, and repeat three times.

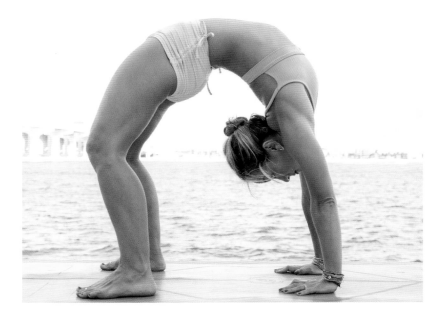

3. *Pinchamayurasana*—Feathered Peacock Pose

Pinchamayurasana is often just called "forearm balance." This pose was a true tapas experience for me. It took me nearly two years of falling over before I found the balance. I remember people telling me they thought I "should" be able to do it already, but I couldn't. I got so frustrated that I considered quitting yoga altogether because I felt I had hit an impenetrable brick wall. But with daily discipline over a sustained period of time, that brick wall started to shift and move. While it seemed like one day I magically caught the balance, it was actually the two years of toppling over when I learned how to balance.

Start in Adho Mukha Svanasana. Exhale as you drop your elbows to the ground. Align your wrists and elbows to avoid a V shape with your arms. Draw your elbows inward to prevent them from splaying out. If you find it difficult to work with precise attention to detail while bearing weight on your arms, you can come down on your knees, adjust your elbows and wrists first, and then stand back up. But if you enter directly from Adho Mukha Svanasana, your hips will already be in place. From the preparation pose, walk your feet forward and stack your hips to align with your shoulders as closely as possible. Engage your shoulder girdle by widening and protracting your shoulders, activating your deltoids and turning on your latissmus dorsi muscles. For the most traditional entry, inhale as you root down through your elbows, send your sacrum forward, pivot through your hips, and lift up into full Pinchamayurasana. If this is not possible, lift one leg while maintaining the power through your shoulder girdle. Avoid overarching your back. Inhale as you lightly jump your hips over the foundation of your arms. Once you find the balance, bring both legs together for the full pose. Gaze at a small point some- where in the space between your thumbs. Stay here for between five and ten breaths.

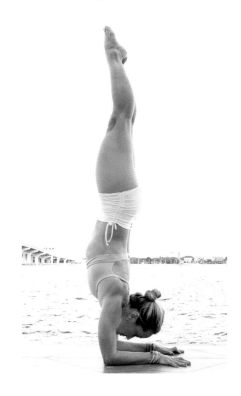

There are many exits from this pose, but for today, just come down in the same manner that you got up, landing softly with as much control as possible. On the exhalation, step back to Chaturanga Dandasana. Inhale and come forward to Urdhva Mukha Svanasana, then exhale and roll back to Adho Mukha Svanasana.

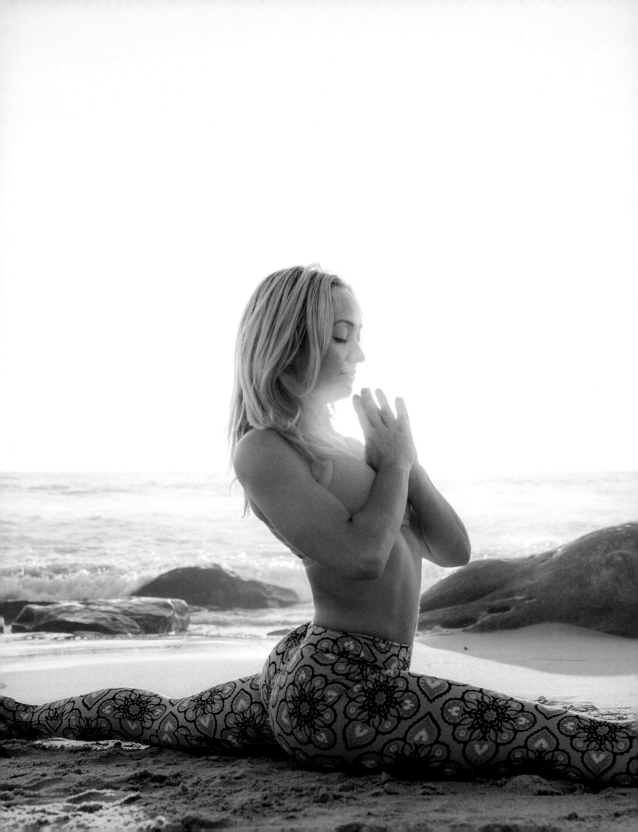

The Crown Jewel of Love
Ratna

Worship of Hanuman is said to bestow all the riches of the world. A legendary figure who is central in the Ramayana and also appears in the Mahabharata, Hanuman is cherished in the Hindu cosmology by many devotees. He represents strength and devotion and the interrelationship between these two facets. The more perfect Hanuman's devotion, the greater his strength. He has the blessings of all the Hindu gods, with each of them giving him either a portion of their powers or protection through their powers. As a student of Surya, the sun god, and son of Pawan, god of wind, Hanuman is presented as an epic hero who accomplishes many impossible tasks, including journeying to the Himalayas to bring back an entire mountain containing an important medicinal root and later leaping across the ocean to Sri Lanka to reunite Rama and Sita.

To be a successful yogi who straddles the dimensions of the physical and material requires great strength and flexibility, much like Hanuman's. Tim Miller, director of the Ashtanga Yoga Center in California and one of the most cherished and respected certified Ashtanga teachers in the world, told me a story about how he could never make a living teaching yoga until Guruji recommended that he place a statue of Hanuman in his yoga shala. Now, I don't personally believe that a statue can bring you wealth and prosperity. But I do believe that everything we achieve is a combination of individual hard work and being receptive to Divine grace. Sometimes after working so hard for so long, we just need to convince ourselves that we are worthy to receive the gracious gift of prosperity.

Today's yogi assignment is gems (*ratna*). Patanjali's Yoga Sutras state that when you release covetousness, the riches of all gems flow to you. *Aparigraha*, the state of noncovetousness, is similar to the state of nonattachment, but it has more to do with nongreed and nonhoarding.

More simply, aparigraha means if you are willing to let go of the need to generate a sense of self-worth through the accumulation of material goods, then you will already have all the wealth you seek.

It is a tricky line to walk, but the key to living in the world as a yogi is to be *in* the world but not *of* it. Define yourself through the eyes of spirit, and root your identity there. Do not let anything in the material world create your sense of self-worth. You are not your car, your job, or the digits in your bank account. You are defined by the kind of person you are when you are having a bad day. You are defined by how much love you share in the world. Place your mind on the riches of the world and you will never be happy, but place your mind on service to God and all riches will flow to you.

When I started yoga, the first thing I did was give away all the accoutrements of my past. I come from an upper-middle-class American family, and I grew up surrounded with every material pleasure and commercial item I ever wanted. But when I read about the *sadhus* and renunciants in yoga, I felt guilty for my material measures; I gave away all my fancy clothes and shoes and designer furniture, traded in my expensive car, shaved my head, replaced jewelry with *malas*, and placed money below morality. While it was a useful period of self-reflection and inner investigation, I realized that I had merely taken on the persona of what I believed a yogi to be. It was not authentically me. I needed to find myself. When I looked inside, I saw that I had big dreams that would require business planning and financial funding. I could not avoid the capitalist framework and live like a total hippie if I wanted to make my dreams come true.

I wanted to make the traditional teaching of yoga available to a large audience. I wanted to inspire millions of people to practice yoga. I wanted to be a worldwide ambassador for yoga as a spiritual path. Along the way, I wanted to open a yoga center, start a clothing line, and build an online portal for yoga videos. And yes, I wanted to be financially successful doing it. People have criticized me for being too material-istic and commercial in the yoga world. People say that I am too vain, too focused on shopping and getting my hair done. Well after having lived the reverse, I can say for sure that I am more myself now than ever before. I am confident and comfortable in the many dimensions of my personality. I love my practice, and I have been devoted to it for more than twenty years, as both a physical practice and a spiritual discipline. But I also embrace the girly side of myself that loves fashion, nails, hair, makeup, and fancy shoes. The difference is that as a yogi, I take responsibility for the choices I make. I do my best to choose vegan fashion and cosmetics, ethically sourced food, and sustainable forms of energy, although I do not always succeed.

I recommend that as a yogi, you reflect on your lifestyle choices rather than buy into anyone's vision of how you should live your life. Whatever you do with a pure heart will succeed, but whatever you do focused solely on financial gain is doomed before it starts. Some sincere yogis block themselves from receiving the riches of the world because they fear the corrupting power of money or identify with a monklike poverty. Perhaps the most important thing is not to get too attached to any material pleasure. At the same time, recognize that success, both spiritual and material, is okay; just be sure you know which one to place at the periphery and which one to place at the core.

1. Define abundance for yourself. What does being rich mean to you? Is it about money, or is it about the quality of love in your life? Are you willing to sacrifice material standards to live a more peaceful life?

2. Put aparigraha into action. Do you hoard clothes or food? Do you let money sit in your bank account unused? Find the place where you have a tendency to save things and tuck them away. Use it or lose it. Either wear the clothes you have or give them away. Eat the stored food or give it away. Invest your money or give a portion to charity.

3. Find the value of love. What does love mean to you? How can love, which is infinite, ever be measured? How can you define what is boundless and knows no end? Think of the love you have shared in your life among family and friends, and try to place a monetary value on it. It is impossible. Recognize that without love, all the riches of the world are vapid, hollow, and meaningless.

PRACTICE   **1.** *Hanumanasana*—Pose Dedicated to Hanuman

The full split is taken from the image of Hanuman's courageous leaps of faith, one from southern India directly to the Himalayas and another from the southernmost tip of India to Sri Lanka. To practice Hanumanasana is much more than to perform the splits. It is an act of service and spiritual strength. It is not enough to be flexible; as a yogi, you must also build the spiritual heart of devotion.

Start in Adho Mukha Svanasana. Inhale as you step your right foot forward. Slide your right leg all the way forward through your arms and settle your hips toward the ground. If your hips do not reach the ground, place a blanket or bolster under them or keep your right leg bent in Anjaneyasana and stay here. Square your hips forward and avoid any tendency to twist or open your pelvis to give the appearance of the pose but sacrifice alignment. Keep your pelvic floor firmly activated, engage your legs, and actively reach out through your toes. The activation is especially important for naturally flexible students. Draw your subnavel in toward your spine, and lift your ribs away from your hips. Avoid arching back too much, and keep your torso aligned over your hips. If you feel ready to proceed deeper, then raise your arms in line with your torso, placing the palms together. Stay here for five breaths.

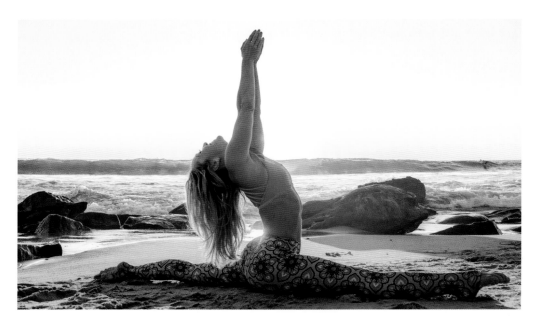

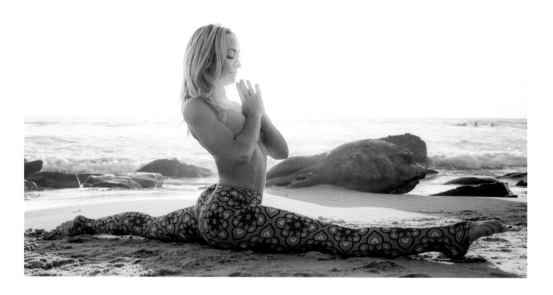

Place your hands in prayer position at the center of your sternum. Stay here for five breaths. Exhale, place your hands on the ground, and step back to Chaturanga Dandasana. Inhale and come forward to Urdhva Mukha Svanasana. Exhale and roll back to Adho Mukha Svanasana. Repeat the pose on the left side.

2. *Trivikramasana*—Standing Splits

Named after Trivikrama, this pose is often just called Standing Splits. Not an easy pose by any means, the name Trivikrama literally means "three" (*tri*) "steps" (*krama*). When you finally enter the full pose, it may feel as epic as the battle between Trivikrama and Bali. You will need strength, flexibility, and equanimity. It took Trivikrama many years before he appeared in front of Bali for the defining moment of the battle for the worlds, so give yourself at least the span of your lifetime to see results.

Start in Samasthiti. Inhale as you raise your right leg and wrap both of your hands around your right foot. If you cannot straighten your leg comfortably or cannot maintain your balance, do not try for the full Trivikramasana. Instead, stay at your limit for five breaths. If you do not feel comfortable approaching this pose, then do Utthita Hasta Padangusthasana.

If you are ready to proceed, inhale as you draw your right leg toward the outer edge of your chest and align your knee with your right armpit. Drop your right hip and avoid hiking the hip too much in order to lift your leg. Drop the head of your right thighbone into its socket to create a stable base. Thrust down through your left leg and straighten your left knee. If possible, lift your right leg all the way up so your whole body stacks along the vertical axis. To deepen Trivikramasana, roll your right shoulder in front of your right thigh, slide your right leg behind the shoulder, and extend your right arm. Gaze upward. Stay here for five breaths, then return to Samasthiti. Repeat on the left side.

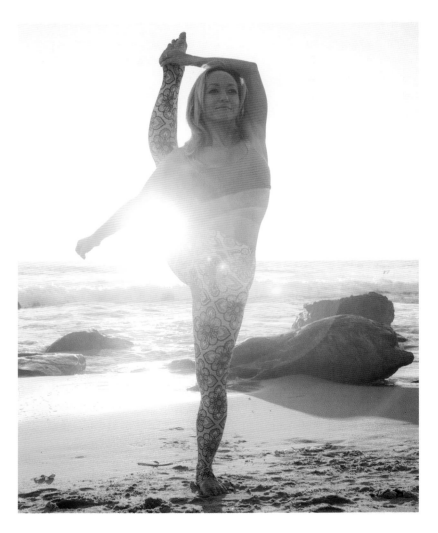

3. *Supta Trivikramasana*—Reclining Splits

This reclining pose is related to the standing splits that bear the same name.

Start off in a supine position. Suck in your lower belly, ground your hips, and press down through your heels. Inhale as you lift your right leg and wrap your hands around your foot. If you cannot straighten your leg comfortably, do not try for the full version of the pose. Instead, stay at your limit for five breaths, or repeat Supta Padangusthasana. Do not use a strap for this pose, just stay where you are and cultivate a devotional attitude of patience.

If you are ready to proceed deeper, inhale as you draw your right leg close to your chest, aligning your right thigh with your right armpit. Ground your left leg by pressing down into your left heel. Point your toes on both feet. Drop the head of your right thighbone deeper into its socket and pull down until your right foot touches the floor. To deepen the pose, roll your right shoulder in front of your right thigh, slide your right leg behind the shoulder, and extend your right arm out to the side. Maintain your left hand's grip on your foot. Gaze toward your nose. Stay here for five breaths. Exhale as you return your right leg to its starting position. Repeat on the left side.

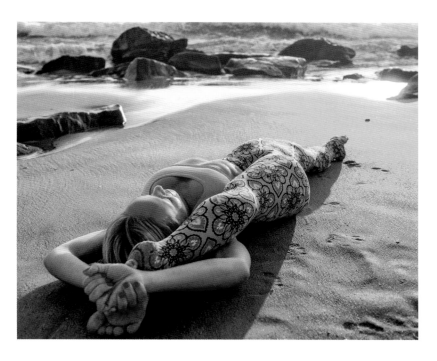

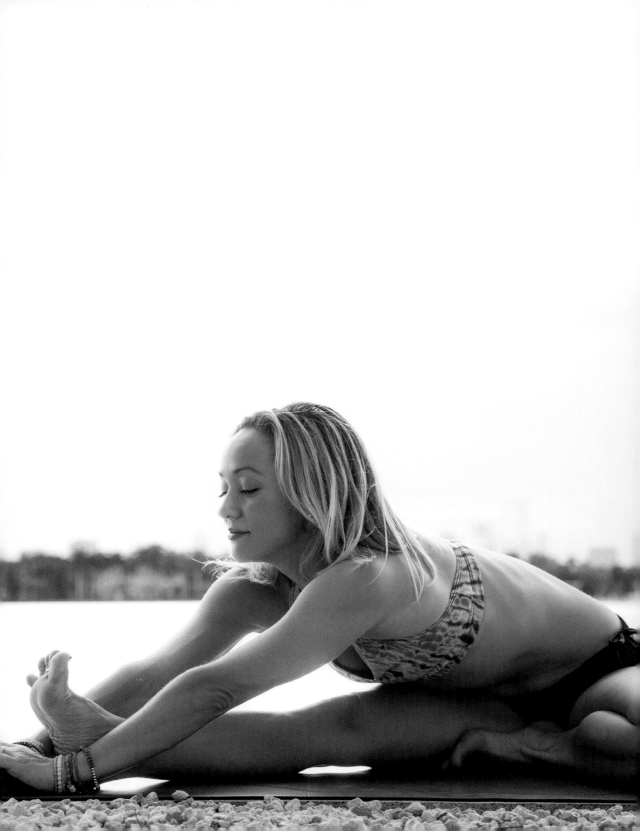

Sacred Space
Mandir

Whether you're in India at an ashram, taking a class at your local yoga center, or practicing on your own at home, to practice is to enter the sacred space—both in terms of physical place and spiritual intention. The word *mandir* signifies a house, temple, or place of worship. It derives from the words *man*, which means inner self, and *dir*, which denotes a dwelling place. Every yoga practice brings you into the sacred space of the inner body. Surrender your emotional defenses and distractions at the altar so you can enter with a humble heart. If you set up your practice space amid text messages, phone calls, social media, and a sea of other distractions, then you are unlikely to truly succeed at journeying away from the material world. Or if you bring your pride, ego, bitterness, jealousy, self-directed negativity, depression, or anger with you onto your yoga mat or into your yoga community, then you have essentially made what is sacred into something profane. Yoga asks you to feel the truth, and once you enter a quiet space of solitude where the inner light dawns, you experience the true self. This liberating experience substantively changes what you value.

Yoga asks the practitioner to look toward a deep inner revelation. What is experienced in a deep yoga practice is often a life-transforming epiphany akin to a sort of peak religious experience. Entering a yoga shala is traditionally like setting foot in a building of worship. Nothing is arranged at random. Instead, each step into the yoga space marks a reorientation from the secular to the spiritual.

In India, at the Ashtanga Yoga Institute, there are many levels of entry that you must pass through before you arrive at the practice space within. The practice space is the heart of the sacred and is physically removed from the noise of secular life. There is a gated entryway that walls off the stairs from the street. Then flanks of stairs lead to a large, carved, wooden double door. Gaining entry through the wooden doors leads you to the marble lobby where you can gaze through a set of carved and decorated wooden doors. In this inner space, bright, colorful carpets line the floor, pictures of important people in the Ashtanga lineage adorn the walls, fresh flowers hang from the altar, and a flame burns at the top of a multitiered golden lamp. Most important, there are more than fifty people there devoting themselves intensively to the inner experience of truth. To say that the energy of the yoga shala in Mysore is palpable is an understatement. Some people call it "Mysore magic," because when you set foot in that shala, all your pains and worries magically go away.

While not every yoga student will travel to India, every yoga student makes the same journey inward with each practice. Today's yogi assignment is sacred space. Ask yourself how you define the sacred, and then perform devotional rituals in service of this highest truth. You might have a home altar or meditation spot dedicated to your spiritual pursuit. It can be as simple or as elaborate as feels right for you. Or you might use the space of your physical body as a holy offering through the vehicle of the practice. The vinyasa method of Ashtanga Yoga ritualizes each breath of the practice to consecrate the body as a worship site. The body itself becomes a sacred space. Or perhaps you have an actual physical location, somewhere in nature, on a remote beach or deep in the mountain woods, that is your place of worship. Or maybe there is a relationship in your life that is sacred to you, a person whose presence calls you forward into your highest truth.

When I hear the opening prayer in the Ashtanga tradition, I always feel a substantive change in the atmosphere, like it has been called forth into spiritual intention. Even just looking at a picture of Guruji makes me think of the sacred space of the practice.

No matter where I am traveling, I always choose a spot for my meditation and yoga practice and claim it as my sacred space. Sunrise, sunset, and the sound of the ocean always bring me to my spiritual home. I have the great blessing of traveling to some of the most beautiful places on earth. I have taught yoga in old churches in Europe, on beaches in Southeast Asia, and in yoga centers all over the world. But one thing that carries through every yoga class is a feeling of the sacred. What makes something spiritual rather than just cultural is the feeling in your heart as you move into the activity. Yoga creates sacred space through the ritual of the practice. With reverence and devotion cultivated from a direct experience of the highest truth, you both honor and create the sacred space of worship in every breath.

1. Create a home altar. Dedicate a space in your home to evoke your sense of the sacred. It can be as simple as a candle or the space of your yoga mat, or as elaborate as an altar table with a picture of your teacher and scared texts that you use for inspiration. Share your intention to create this sacred space with your family or housemates, and include them in the process so they respect and understand your decision to create an altar.

2. Honor sacred space. Visit a yoga center, church, temple, or other place of worship. Pay careful attention to the details, including the architecture, geometry, and sites of prayer, meditation, or practice. Reflect on how the organization of the space creates a sense of the sacred.

3. Consecrate the sacred space of your body. Through the vinyasa method of coordinating breath to movement, the yoga practitioner is invited to consecrate the inner space of the body. Perform this action with heightened inner awareness. Drop your mind deep within the inner body, and scan through your body, leaving no muscle or cell unseen. Bathe your body with the light of inner awareness, and reveal the sacred space of the inner body.

1. *Adho Mukha Svanasana*—Downward-Facing Dog Pose

One of the fundamental poses of all yoga styles, Adho Mukha Svanasana is not as easy as it may first appear. To enter the pose, it's traditional to simply roll back from Urdhva Mukha Svanasana. However, if you are newer to the practice, start off on your hands and knees. Place your hands shoulder-width apart and your feet hip-width apart. Curl your toes under, draw your subnavel toward your spine, and send your hips back and up to enter Adho Mukha Svanasana.

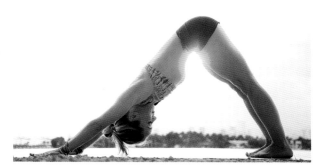

Rotate your shoulder joints outward to spread your shoulder blades. Avoid sinking too far into your shoulders and actively reach outward through your fingertips. Pivot from your hip joints, allowing them to flex deeply. Straighten your legs as much as possible. Engage your quadriceps and root down through the bases of your big toes. Tuck your chin under and gaze toward your navel. Stay here for five breaths. Then exhale and come down to Balasana to rest.

Adho Mukha Svanasana is a kind of home because it is used so often as a resting point in the practice. Turning the mind inward to the sensation of the sacred space of the inner body draws your attention deeper and invites a more meditative approach to the practice.

2. Janu Sirsasana A—Head-to-Knee Pose

Start in Dandasana. Exhale as you draw your left knee in toward your chest to close the knee joint. Drop your left knee out to the side by

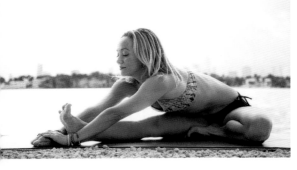

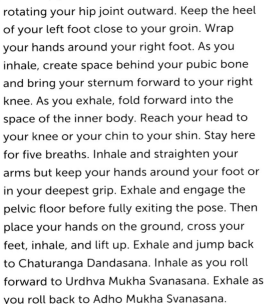

rotating your hip joint outward. Keep the heel of your left foot close to your groin. Wrap your hands around your right foot. As you inhale, create space behind your pubic bone and bring your sternum forward to your right knee. As you exhale, fold forward into the space of the inner body. Reach your head to your knee or your chin to your shin. Stay here for five breaths. Inhale and straighten your arms but keep your hands around your foot or in your deepest grip. Exhale and engage the pelvic floor before fully exiting the pose. Then place your hands on the ground, cross your feet, inhale, and lift up. Exhale and jump back to Chaturanga Dandasana. Inhale as you roll forward to Urdhva Mukha Svanasana. Exhale as you roll back to Adho Mukha Svanasana.

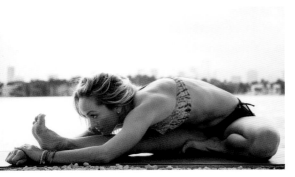

The meditative state of calm equipoise allows you to access your core muscles, hollow out your pelvic bowl, and create space behind your pubic bone. A deceptively simple pose, Janu Sirsasana A gives you access to the sacred space of the inner body.

3. *Vrksasana*—Tree Pose

What appears at first to be a simple standing pose builds the foundation of deeper awareness in the practice and ultimately within yourself. Like the threshold to the sacred spaces of yoga shalas, Vrksasana helps you plant the roots of spiritual practice.

Start in Samasthiti. Inhale as you roll your right hip outward, bend the knee, and draw your right foot up along the inner edge of your left leg. If your balance is challenged, rest your right foot along your lower leg. If possible, slide the foot all the way toward your groin. Press your right foot firmly against your left inner thigh and create a kind of bind between the two. Draw your subnavel in toward your spine, and lift your ribs away from your hips while tucking in your lower ribs. Join your hands in prayer position, and gaze at your nose. Stay here for five breaths. Exhale and lower your leg. Repeat on the left side.

This may, at first, seem like a simple pose, but there is great depth available to you in Vrksasana. As a balancing pose, it trains the mind and body to maintain a solid center line. One of the deepest yogic states happens when the mind and body are drawn in toward this place of equanimity in the inner body. A seemingly simple pose like Vrksasana makes the illusive inner state of equanimity accessible to many practitioners.

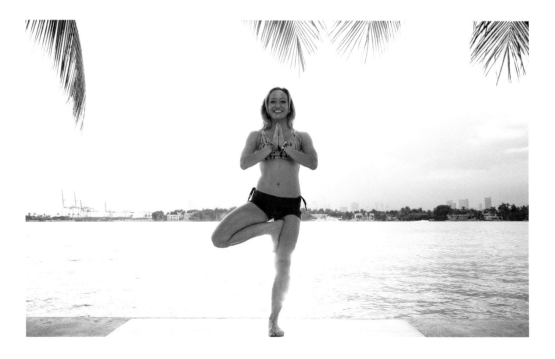

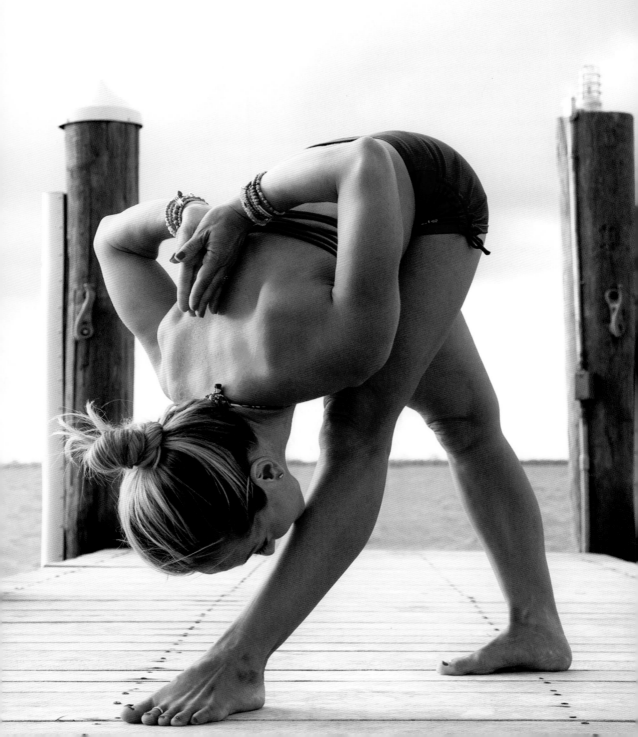

You Are Worthy
Purusa

have faced periods of great sorrow and been crippled with doubt and depression. Out of desperation, I ran from my sadness and hit the bottom of the sea of my own consciousness. But there is wisdom in sadness, truth in sorrow. Cheerfulness is lovely, like a spring blossom. But winter brings its own revelations. If there is one thing I've learned from the practice of yoga, it's not to run from pain. Your pain is your greatest teacher. The cracks in the cheerfulness filter on your life are actually your greatest asset. Sorrow brings earnestness, longing, justice, and compassion. Doubt can lead you to humility, true self-confidence, and even a return to innocence. There is beauty and grace in sadness. Like the winter, periods of apparent suffering are often important times of growth, resetting your inner clock to a time zone closer to your spiritual home.

If you are suffering right now, don't run and don't give up. Instead, dig in, dive deep, and just experience it, get comfortable with it. Make friends with your tears and let them be your teacher. Let the search for meaning guide to you a new spiritual lesson, and see the truth revealed through your trials and tribulations. It's there, hiding in the fragility of a raindrop and the perfection of a snowflake, the hidden meaning of it all, so simple and yet totally complex, perfectly whole but glimmering in a thousand little pieces of love.

Yoga can sometimes be difficult and demanding. The practice asks you to face your pain and make no pretense of strength where you have none. Expose the raw truth of your unedited self. Leave nothing hidden and keep nothing tucked away in a dark corner of the mind. See clearly through the mirror of life reflected back to you in your actions, thoughts, and deeds. Everyone who commits to the sincere practice of yoga has experienced the nearly intangible, ineffable realm of the spirit. It is not the poses that heal, nor is it the technique that liberates.

Instead, yoga is a bridge of experience. The subtlety of the spirit cannot be intellectualized, but it can be felt through the channel of the heart. It is most often pain and suffering that crack the surface level of personality just enough to let the spirit shine through.

Today's yogi assignment is spirit (*purusa*). The whole path of yoga can be understood as a vehicle for you to experience your true nature, or purusa. The dichotomy between purusa (the eternal, whole, perfect spirit within every sentient being) and *prakrti* (material reality) forms the fundamental power struggle in the yogi's battle. There is a choice between the eternal and the temporal, the singular and the multiple, the changeless and the impermanent, and the noumenal and the phenomenal. Traditionally, both purusa and prakrti are considered to be divinely created and eternal. Somewhere along the timeline of history, we misidentified ourselves in the world of form and function and forgot our essence as pure spirit. Essentially, we forgot who we really are. The practice of yoga teaches you how to orient every breath in your practice, and ultimately every choice in your life, in your identity as purusa. In many ways, yoga can be seen as an awakening of the true light within, that true light being the eternal presence of spirit.

Seeking permanence in the world of prakrti is hitting an emotional and spiritual rock bottom. When you realize that permanent happiness cannot be found in the material world, you will also see that you are not defined by your possessions or accomplishments, on or off the yoga mat. The best thing about the sorrow of the world, your sorrow and pain, is that it leads you to yearn for a permanent sense of self, a happiness that never fades. Yoga teaches you to sit with your sorrow because it will soften your heart and lead you into an experience in the realm of purusa. Once you define yourself in terms of the eternal Divine spark that rests in your inner being, that truth will literally set you free. Define yourself by worldly attachments, achievements, or accomplishments and you will always find yourself hungry, desperate, and lost.

Without any direct experience of purusa, you will doubt your intrinsic worth and always feel like something is lacking. The irony is that those who are hardest on themselves are often the most worthy; they just don't see the plain truth that is evident to everyone else. Yoga helps you counter these negative feelings by planting the seed of faith. You don't have to earn your worthiness to be loved. It is quite literally your spiritual inheritance. In other words, your basic worthiness comes from the essence of your spirit. You are born with it, and you don't need to do anything to get it. You just have to realize who you really are and let all the love in. If, in your heart, you carry the burden of not feeling good enough, either you will internalize the feeling of unworthiness and end up depressed or anxious and blame yourself, or you will externalize it and end up in a mad dash for worldly success and blame the world. Either way, sooner or later, the glass house of identifying solely with prakrti will come crashing down. It is through faith alone that you realize your worthiness and can be free of that darkness. While pain and sorrow are not fun, it is the difficult experiences that create the fertile ground of a receptive heart so you can plant the seed of faith within yourself. You are worthy not because of anything you have done but because your true nature is in the spirit.

But what exactly does it feel like to set your mind free from its entanglement in the material world and reorient your sense of identity in the spirit? Perhaps purusa defies our ability to describe it because it is ultimately not of this world of mind and matter, it is not and cannot be bound by words and logic. Even the great sage Patanjali chose not to answer that question. Accordingly to him, the final state of liberation happens when purusa recognizes its true nature and never wavers from that state, but he leaves the question of what that actually feels like unanswered. There is no great flowering poem about Divine revelation, no attempt to define the eternal realm of the spirit in the Yoga Sutras. There is only the technique that will lead you to the experience firsthand. Yoga is a practice more than a philosophy. It is an experiential tool whose efficacy rests in the ability of the practitioner to directly perceive the most rarefied states of the spirit within. Every step along the yoga path is a movement deeper into the realization of purusa.

Since you're reading this book, you have probably already experienced the Divine elixir of the eternal and that is why you practice yoga. You have perhaps had a flash, like an epiphany or a peak experience, that left you forever changed. You may have gotten a glimpse of the spirit in a practice so deep and mind-altering that your world has never been quite the same. You may have felt the presence of an imperturbable peace, a limitless compassion, or a deep sense of purpose. Or maybe you have simply been filled with the resplendent emptiness of timelessness, a beingness so pure that it shines and overtakes you like a lightning bolt, knocks you out cold, so that you finally wake up to the truth of who you are and see yourself though the eyes of the spirit.

HOMEWORK

1. Reflect. Sit with your sorrow and don't fight it. Just observe. Make peace with what you feel. Think back on a time of difficulty. Observe the lesson you learned and how it has shaped who you are and what you value. With an open, humble heart, ask what the lesson from your suffering is. Be willing to learn and hear the answer. What changes did you make as a result of the revelations afforded to you after the period of suffering?

2. Think about the presence of spirit. Think of a time when you felt the presence of spirit. Perhaps it is in a piece of music, a piece of artwork, or a dramatic performance that you loved. Or perhaps it is in a recent yoga practice during which you were powerfully moved by the spirit within. While it may be difficult, see if you can define what it was about these moments that brought you in touch with the ineffable spirit.

3. Find spiritual motivation. What is the spiritual motivation that guides all your actions? Rather than searching outside yourself to achieve, relocate your point of identity to the spirit within. Then allow all your actions to flow from this inexhaustible source.

PRACTICE

1. *Parsvottanasana*—Intense Side Stretch Pose

Start in Samasthiti. Hold your elbows behind your back. If this is comfortable, press your fingertips together in the small of your back and glide your hands into prayer position. Placing your hands in prayer position behind your back can be thought of as a symbol of reverence toward the spiritual world that is so often out of sight but clearly felt. Inhale as you step out to the right, leaving a distance slightly shorter than one leg-length between your feet. This distance is adjustable based on your height, leg length, and level of flexibility. Pivot on your feet and square your hips to the back of your mat. Turn your left foot out forty-five degrees by gently rotating your left hip outward. Align your left heel with your right arch. Suck in your subnavel to create space. Exhale as you fold forward. Send your sternum forward toward the inner edge of your left knee. Allow your sternum, left knee, and

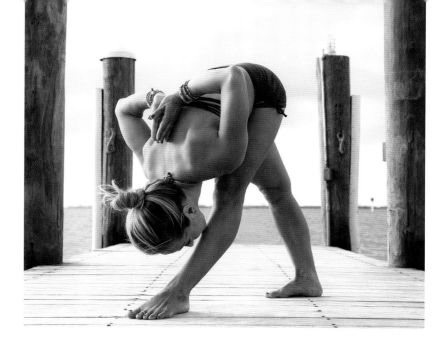

pubic bone to line up along the central axis. Pivot from your hips as you fold forward and distribute your weight evenly between your two legs. Avoid rounding your back too much, but do not arch your spine or keep it rigid. Drop your head and reach your nose or the top of your head to your left knee, eventually reaching your chin forward to your shin. Gaze either at your nose or your left foot. Keep your pelvic floor engaged. With equal strength, draw in your subnavel to create space behind your pubic bone and elongate your hamstrings and lower back as you fold forward. Stay here for five breaths.

Inhale as you lift your torso by pivoting through your hips and sending your pubic bone up and forward. Turn on the balls of your feet, keep your hands in position, and repeat on the right side. After five breaths on the right side, inhale as you come up and return to Samasthiti.

2. Mukta Hasta Sirsasana A—Tripod Headstand

All inversions powerfully plug you into the center line of the body and Mukta Hasta Sirsasana A tests both mental and physical strength. This first of the unsupported headstands is a shoulder and core strengthener. Without the support of the elbows on the ground, as in the more common Baddha Hasta Sirsasana series, Mukta Hasta Sirsasana A often brings up fear about stabilizing the neck. Yet with a little technique, this headstand can be made accessible to all. You just need a little bit of faith.

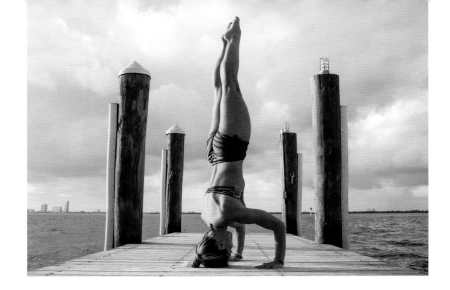

Start off on your hands and knees. Exhale as you place the top of your head on the ground in front of your fingertips to form a tripod base between your two palms and your head. Make sure the flattest point at the very top of your head is on the ground. Avoid rolling forward on your forehead or keeping your weight toward the back of your head. Engage your shoulder girdle and stabilize your arms. Align your elbows above your wrists and keep them bent at ninety-degree angles. Inhale as you stand your legs up and walk forward toward your arms. If your balance or strength feels challenged, stay in this preparatory position for five breaths and then come down.

If you are ready to progress, inhale as you pivot your hips forward over the solid foundation of your arms to lift up. Do not attempt to jump up or kick one leg up into Mukta Hasta Sirsasana A. If you cannot lift up in a pike position, bend your knees and walk your knees into the armpits to climb up. If you maintain a good balance with your knees bent, inhale and straighten your legs up from there. Draw in your lower ribs, stabilize your shoulder girdle, tuck your tailbone slightly, engage your quadriceps, and point your toes. Gaze at the tip of your nose. Stay here for five breaths. Come down in the same manner as you lifted up. Rest in Balasana for five breaths.

Note that it is not recommended to hold Mukta Hasta Sirsasana A for sustained periods of time due to the unsupported nature of the pose. As your strength grows, you can use this pose as the base for many challenging arm balances. Think of the strength and stability cultivated in Mukta Hasta Sirsasana A as a metaphor for the spiritual foundation for all of life's activities.

3. *Matsyasana*—Fish Pose

Named after Matsya, the avatar of the Hindu god Vishnu, who appears in the form of a fish, Matsyasana is included in the Ashtanga Yoga Closing Poses to integrate the deep lessons of backbending and strengthen the spine. Matsya rescues the first man, Manu, from an epic flood not unlike the story of Noah's ark. Symbolic of salvation, Matsya appears in numerous stories as the incarnation of God to guide the human Manu to safety or righteous action. Surrender is a key component in any backbend, but in Matsyasana, it is balanced by inner strength.

Start in Padmasana. If you cannot access this pose, straighten your legs and point your toes. Use your elbows to lift your torso and arch your spine. Roll back through your neck and extend your cervical spine and lower your head to the ground. Draw in your subnavel and pivot your sacrum forward into nutation, drawing it forward and slightly up into the pelvis. If you are in Padmasana, hold the tops of your feet and straighten your elbows. If your knees feel good, reach them toward the ground, but avoid putting any unnecessary strain on your joints. If your legs are straight, place your hands next to your hips and leave your elbows resting on the ground. Gaze at the space between your eyebrows, known as the *ajna* chakra, or third eye center. Stay here for eight to ten breaths. Then slowly release to a supine position; if you are in Padmasana, straighten your legs.

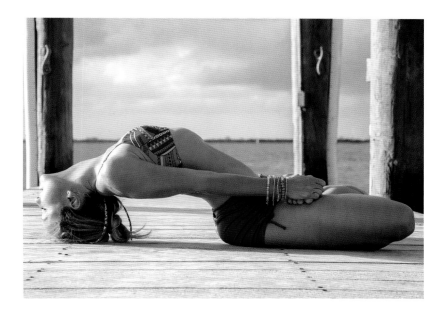

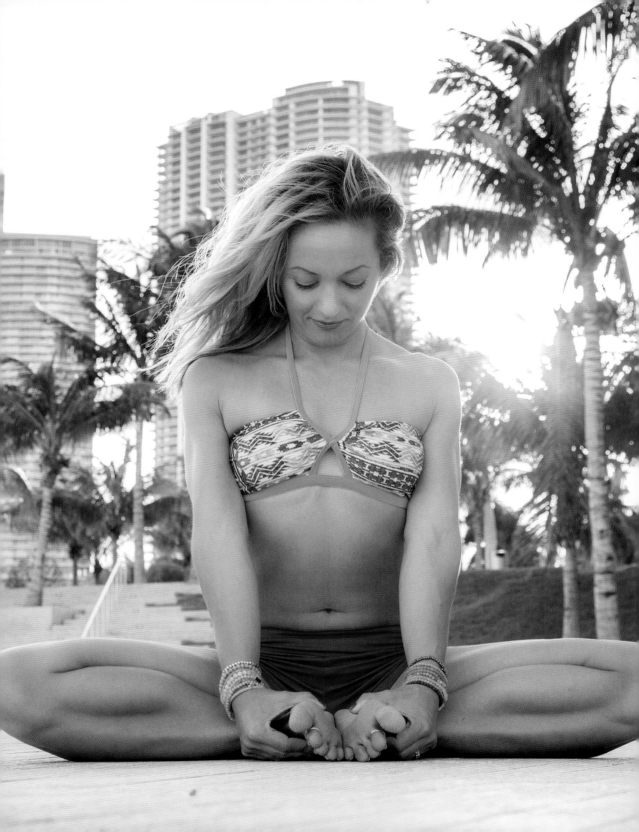

Day 26 | Yoga as a Personal Practice
Abhyasa

The single most defining factor in establishing your practice is your commitment to unroll your mat every day. Whether you are practicing under the supervision of a teacher or on your own, it is your decision to make the practice a part of your life. The truth about yoga is that it is all too often a solitary journey. There are lonely, dark mornings when you have to drag yourself to your mat. There are days with little inspiration and overwhelming monotony, and a lot of stiff days when everything hurts. But still you practice. And there are certainly days when you float in the clouds, when everything bends and the sun is shining. On those glorious days, you relish your practice. But you practice every day.

Practice is a daily devotional ritual that, once integrated into your routine, is something that just becomes part of who you are. Once an activity is ritualized, it happens around the same time every day and requires little effort to maintain. Not that practice will be easy, but once you have an established personal practice, it won't feel so hard to actually get on your mat. Just like you brush your teeth every day even if you are tired, sore, sleepy, or traveling, you practice no matter where you are or how you feel. In this way, practice is simply a part of your life.

Today's yogi assignment is practice (*abhyasa*). Yoga is a personal practice focused sincerely on spiritual realization. While practice may take many external forms, the deeper intention remains the same. It doesn't have to be an Olympic-level expression of physical prowess, although it could be. It could also take the form of sitting meditation or a healing, restorative practice. Patanjali provides three foundational elements of practice in Yoga Sutra 1.14. Practice attains a firm ground (*dridha bhumih*) when it is done over a long time (*dirgha kala*), such as one human lifetime; without a break (*nairantarya*); and with sincerity, devotion, and reverence (*satkara*). It takes both strength and patience to embark on the long road of yoga and be willing to work for your entire life to attain the results of inner peace.

The commitment to practice without a break means both to practice every day and to keep the moral and ethical principles of the yoga path in your heart at all times. Finally, your intention is perhaps the most defining factor in the ultimate success of your practice. If your heart is invested in the deeper spiritual goals of yoga, then any little effort you exert in your asana practice will reap immense rewards. Attaining firm ground and dutifully applying these three elements to your practice are a daunting task that requires concerted effort.

Ideally, practice happens at the same time every day and on the same days each week. Your body responds well to routine, so practicing at the same time helps you optimize your practice. Like a clock that helps set your inner rhythms, practicing at the same time every day also helps improve digestion and restful sleep. Asana practice is best done under the guidance of a teacher so that you have a set program to follow and are not left standing on your mat wondering what to do. Too many yogis fall off the program of practice because they are their own teachers and get lost, injured, or distracted when they have to create their own routine. Every top-level athlete has a coach and a trainer, and every yogi preferably has a teacher who helps them set their practice program. At the same time, you are the one who has to put in the work. The teacher or trainer can only do so much. Some students never practice unless their teacher is watching or they go to class. To be truly transformational, the practice must ultimately be yours. While I travel to India once a year to spend time with my teacher, most of my time on the mat is spent alone.

According to Yoga Sutra 1.22, there are three levels of yoga practitioners: mild (*mrdu*), medium (*madhya*), and intense (*adhimatratvat*). All three levels will eventually succeed on the yoga journey. We will all vacillate between the three categories over the course of our lives. There is no need to be intense all the time and force yourself to rush toward eternity. It is, after all, eternity and therefore will be exactly the same if you experience it today, tomorrow, next year, or in ten thousand years. Guruji's simple words are absolutely true: "Practice, practice, practice, and all is coming."

Only by fully releasing your need to get anywhere at any particular time does the power of practice really start to take effect. There is a humility that can only be cultivated over years of getting on the mat and putting in the work with no attachment to the goal. You have to learn to hear that quiet voice in your heart that says, *I will stay the course and keep the faith no matter how long it takes.* Yoga is a personal practice.

Only you can choose to turn your mind inward and experience the deepest truth. No one can walk your path for you. Unroll the mat and practice for many years, with a sincere heart and an undaunted spirit.

Some days, I feel like a hero for even getting on my mat. Sometimes I crawl to it for a very lazy, sleepy Primary Series. Sometimes I cannot wait to get on my mat and practice. Some days, I feel like I am flying, but most days, I am just putting in the work. Practice does not need to be perfect; you just need to do it. The most important part of practice is that you do it every day. Get on your mat, because even five minutes have the power to change your day, clear out troubling emotions, and set your intention to live a more peaceful life.

HOMEWORK

1. If you have a mild-level practice. There is no substitute for getting on your mat. Commit yourself to practicing for at least five minutes every day for the next month. A good program would be six days a week of asana practice and one day a week of meditation. Let go of all attachment to any postural goals and focus instead on the steady commitment to maintain the spiritual discipline of a personal practice for thirty consecutive days. Keep a practice journal to log your practice time and keep track of your progress.

2. If you have a medium-level practice. Increase the intensity of your practice by adding time to your abhyasa. Commit yourself to a minimum of twenty minutes of daily practice for one month. Remember to include one day a week of meditation to give your body time to rest and recover from the increased intensity of the physical discipline. Follow the guidelines outlined in Day Nine for instructions and guidelines on how to meditate.

3. If you have an intense practice. Commit yourself to doing a minimum of one full hour of practice six days a week. Take one day off from any physical activity and focus on meditation. At this point, yoga will change your life. Practicing for at least sixty minutes a day has a substantive impact on your schedule and gently encourages you to make the lifestyle changes that a yogi's life requires. Once you integrate a minimum of one hour of physical discipline into your day, yoga starts to take over your life in the best possible way. It will be hard to take a day off because you will feel a void on the days when you don't practice. In this state of abhyasa, it is crucial to integrate one day off of physical practice per week. Honoring the day of physical rest is another form of nonattachment and prevents you from developing an unhealthy attachment to the intensity of asana. You can maintain nairantarya by developing your meditation practice on the rest day.

PRACTICE

1. *Baddha Konasana*—Bound Angle Pose

To succeed at Baddha Konasana—also known as Cobbler's Pose—with a calm and equanimous mind, you will need equal parts practice and nonattachment. If you set your mind on the physical goal of "getting your knees down," you may sacrifice both your physical health and your spiritual journey for a hollow goal. Instead, release all attachment to the physical shape and focus on the inner body. Do not be surprised if this pose takes years to feel good, regardless of how well you do other poses in the practice.

Start in Dandasana. Tune in to your hip joints as you engage your pelvic floor. Draw your knees in toward your chest to close your knee joints. Exhale as you rotate your hips outward and allow your knees to descend toward the ground. Draw your heels in as close to your groin as possible. Hold on to the bases of your big toes, and open the soles of your feet upward. Tuck your chin, or gaze at your feet (see photo).

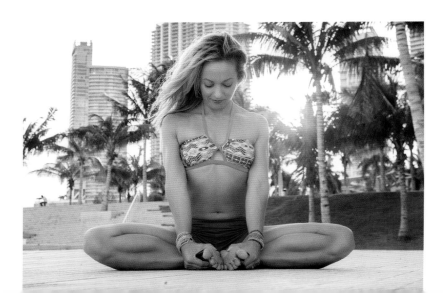

Exhale as you pivot your pubic bone and sitting bones back to fold forward from your hip joints. Keep your spine as straight as possible and your subnavel drawn back toward your spine. Once you reach your maximum forward bend, allow the top of your head, your nose, or your chin to touch the ground, depending on your level of flexibility. Your hands remain on your feet. Avoid pushing on your knees and simply accept where you are. Stay here for five to ten breaths. Inhale as you come up, straighten your legs, and return to Dandasana.

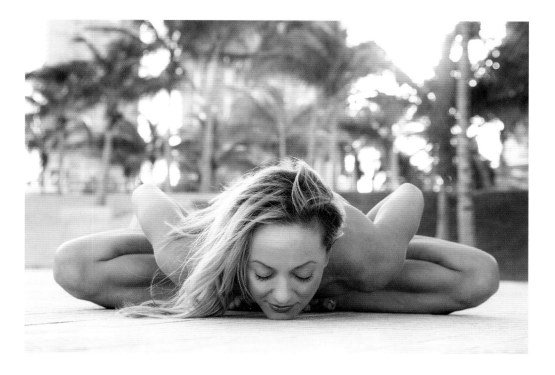

2. Navasana—Boat Pose

Perhaps no other pose illustrates the need to practice as clearly as Navasana. It requires a strong and steady mind and the commitment to practice. It is the only pose in the Ashtanga Yoga method that is repeated five times in a row. The repetition itself is emblematic of the consistent effort that true practice demands.

Start in Dandasana. Inhale as you lean slightly back through your hips, rolling your pelvis down to the space between your sitting bones and tailbone. Lift your legs as you send your torso slightly back to counterbalance. Draw in your lower belly, and engage your lower abdominal muscles, pelvic floor, and core muscles. Keep your toes pointed and your legs together. Straighten your arms in front of you at shoulder-height. Straighten your legs as much as possible, but avoid rounding your back and sinking too close to the ground to do this. Keep your body relatively upright; your torso and thighs should form about an eighty-degree angle. Gaze toward your toes. Stay here for five breaths. Repeat five times.

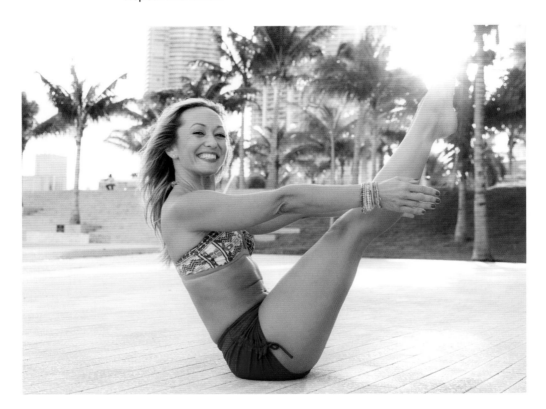

3. *Shalabhasana*—Locust Pose

This humble backbend is very much like the practice itself, founded on steady perseverance over a long time. It is not to be confused with the contemporary yoga pose called Grasshopper Pose. Rather than trying to achieve the deepest backbend, Shalabhasana is about endurance and strength over the long haul. It is often used as a therapeutic backbend to treat herniated discs and other back issues. Putting the foundational work into Shalabhasana sets up your practice well for backbends from both the physical and the spiritual paradigm.

Start off lying on your stomach. Place your hands next to your hips, keep your arms straight, and turn your palms up. Inhale as you draw in your subnavel, tilt the sacrum slightly up and into the pelvis, engage your quadriceps, and lift your legs. Simultaneously, send your sternum forward and lift your chest, but keep your lower ribs on the ground. Reach your sternum forward and slightly up while you extend your legs back and slightly up. Avoid bending your knees to lift your feet higher; instead, lengthen your body and maximize the space between your vertebrae. Gaze at your nose. Stay here for five breaths.

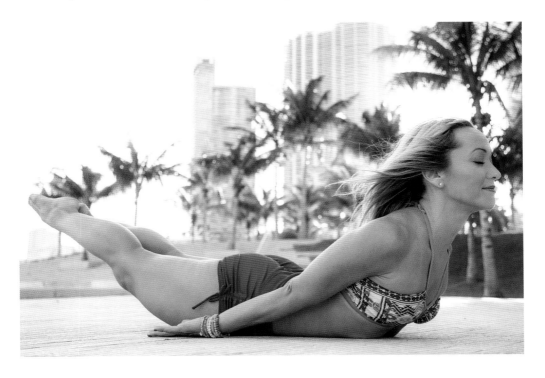

If you feel fatigued, exhale and come down, pull your knees into your chest, and rest in Balasana. Or, if you feel energized, inhale directly into Urdhva Mukha Svanasana; exhale and roll back to Adho Mukha Svanasana.

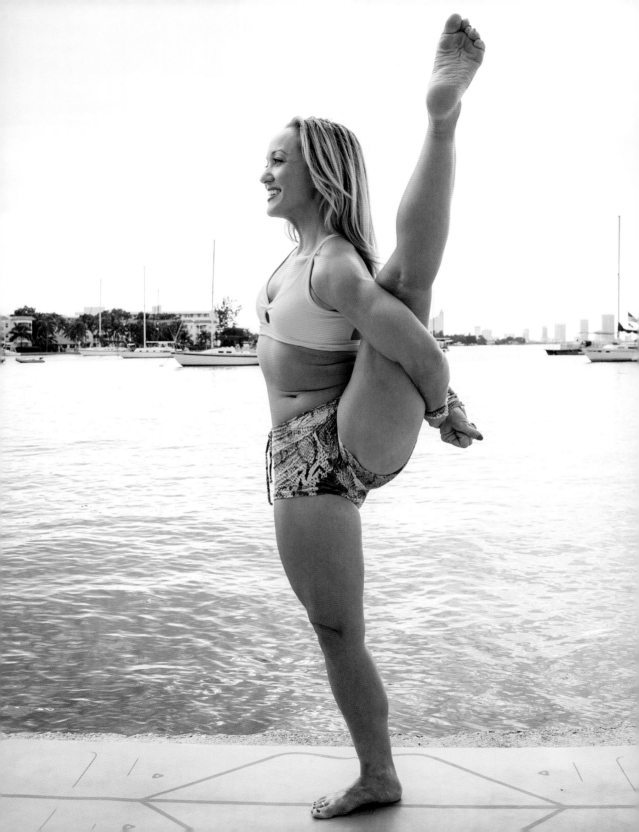

Letting Go and Letting God
Vairagya

'm a fighter, tenacious to a fault. I don't walk away, back down, or quit. I can also be rebellious, willful, and stubborn. Yoga has taught me that sometimes walking away is the strongest and bravest thing you can do. I remember trying an arm balance fifteen times in a row, demanding that my body get into the pose. People suggested that I stop, but I kept going. I never asked my body how it felt or what it wanted to do. I just plowed on. It didn't serve me well or make the pose happen. I got tired and exhausted, and I was left feeling defeated. Then one day, another path opened to me; instead of fighting for the poses, I could ease my way into them. All it took was surrender. As soon as I let go of my attachment to doing the pose that day or any day, I suddenly had space to listen to my body. Instead of forcing my way through blindly, I could wait for inner guidance and follow the path that was presented.

How many times have you heard a voice offering gentle guidance only to turn away from it in favor of your personal preference? How many times have you heard your body ask for mercy, but you push through and end up in pain? Listening to the inner voice of wisdom also comes with a responsibility to follow the path as it is revealed to you. Today's yogi assignment is nonattachment (*vairagya*). Patanjali states in Yoga Sutra 1.12 that practice (abhyasa) must be balanced with the element of nonattachment (vairagya) to achieve its goal of a peaceful mind (nirodah).

Without balance between practice and nonattachment, the mind will tend to obsess about the aesthetic shape of the body and may get overly attached to the body. You may end up judging your success by whether or not you are able to attain the perfect form of a yoga pose and sub-jecting your body to harsh treatment to attain that pose. But yoga seeks to free your mind from attachment to the physical form and root your identity at the spirit level within. Only with practice and nonattachment will you achieve the equanimous mind that is the essence of yoga. The only way you really can let go of your individual will is to trust that there is a Divine will that is greater and working in your best interest. In other words, you need to have the faith to let go and turn it over to a God.

Guruji always recommended that students read the epic story of the Bhagavad Gita, in which the warrior prince Arjuna receives the teaching of yoga from Krishna on the eve of a decisive battle between two warring factions. *Vairagya* literally means "without emotion or interest." But applied in a yogic context, it usually means "without attachment to the fruits of one's labor." Krishna explains to Arjuna in the Gita 6.35 that only with abhyasa and vairagya will the restless mind become steady and calm. Echoing Patanjali's definition of nonattachment paired with practice as the path to inner calm, Krishna offers a more concrete understanding of exactly how to let go of the passionate attachment to one's own life goals. He offers himself as the vehicle for nonattachment. He explains that Arjuna is to trust God's will and surrender the fruits of his labor to God.

Another way to understand the pairing of practice and nonattachment is to recognize that when we attain the fruits of our labor through our will, it builds the ego. In that scenario, what we attain only ensnares us further in the cycle of suffering. But when we work and surrender the fruits of our labor to God, we are free from the "I" in our success. In other words, yogis work and work over many years of consistent practice with the sober and humble recognition that all we attain comes from the grace of God. And from the act of surrendering our individual will to Divine will comes lasting peace and ultimate freedom.

You can either operate from this deep place of connection or try to do it all yourself. You can use force, apply pressure, compete with yourself and others, fight, claw, dramatize, react, antagonize, and rant. You can waste time worrying and stressing, but no amount of worrying will ever change a situation, and no amount of stressing ever solved a problem. Thinking that you can control all the details of the grand orchestra of life is a false hubris that will eventually result in cacophony rather than a symphony. Instead of trying to be in control, surrender. Let tomorrow worry about tomorrow; keep your mind and heart present today. As long as you're operating from the mind-set that you have to hold all the pieces of your life together, you're blocking yourself from receiving the biggest gift of all—grace. Don't sweat the small stuff or the big stuff. Leave sweating for the yoga mat, and enjoy your life. No matter what happens, don't worry. If you miss a flight, flunk a test, get fired, get sick, have your heart broken, go bankrupt, get injured, get bad news, suffer loss of any kind—don't worry, it will all be okay. You are okay.

You can choose to operate in trust and surrender, or you will find yourself caught by the snares of fear and control. Yoga is not built on theory alone, so just for today, trust. Try it out. Heal past betrayals that have wounded your heart. Cast out grudges and be brave enough to believe again. Just for today, surrender. Feel the ease and flow that come when the burden of stress and anxiety lifts off your heart. Wait for it. Because the blessings of more peace and happiness than you ever thought possible are coming just for you. All you need to do is trust and surrender.

1. Let go and let God. Is there some place in your life where you feel blocked? Are you trying to force your will on a situation? Is something stressing you out, and you can't stop worrying about it? Meditate for at least five minutes. Write down your desire and then surrender the fruits of your labor—that is, your desired outcome. Turn it over to God, and let it go. Trust that if it is meant to be, it will be. But if it's not meant to be, then you will be blessed by the desire not manifesting.

HOMEWORK

2. Keep track of the real goal. Take time each day to remember the simple things. Love is what matters. Sunrise, sunset, ocean, and sky. This is the breath of life. Breathe deeply. Nothing matters because you already have everything in your heart. You are whole and complete.

3. Conduct an empirical test. For one twenty-four-hour period, don't plan anything. Wake up and see where you are guided. Go one full day without a to-do list and then evaluate if you felt happier and more free. You may fear that if you don't plan out your day and control all the details, nothing will get done, but just try it and see what happens. Did the world fall apart without your plan? Were there maybe a few more moments of spontaneity and love? It's hard to schedule in happiness, love, laughter, and joy. Instead, let go of the need to control and let it all flow into your life.

PRACTICE

1. *Utthan Pristhasana*—Lizard Pose

This pose is a great place to work on flexibility in your hips. *Utthan* is usually translated as "stretch out," but it can also mean regeneration. Citing the regenerative qualities of the lizard, the traditional Sanskrit speaks to the lesson contained within this pose. Hips often get tight from long car rides, stress, or general stiffness. Just as the lizard is happy to let go of its tail and grow a new one, so must you let go of all the tightness in your hips and open your body and mind to new levels of freedom. *Pristha* can mean the pages of a book, so you can also think of opening your hips like opening the book of your pelvis wide.

There are many variations of Utthan Pristhasana, so let's begin with one of the most accessible. Start in Adho Mukha Svanasana. Inhale as you step your left foot forward. Exhale as you plant your right knee on the ground. Drop your right hip, and draw your left thigh toward your chest. Inhale as you extend your left arm and drop your right hand to the ground for additional support. Look up to the fingertips of your left hand. Stay here for five breaths. Exhale, return both hands to the ground, and step back to Chaturanga Dandasana. Inhale and roll forward to Urdhva Mukha Svanasana. Exhale and roll back to Adho Mukha Svanasana. Repeat on the right side.

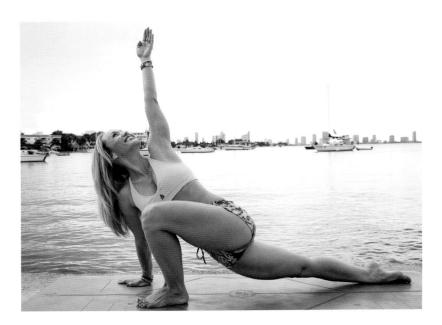

2. Svarga Dvijasana—Bird of Paradise Pose

This elegant pose takes a lot of practice. *Dvija* means "twice born," and *svarga* means "paradise" or "heaven." Most of people need more than a few tries before they feel like they are ascending to heaven. Instead, they may feel more like the flower bud that requires patience, nurturance, and kindness to come to full bloom. Before you attempt this pose, be sure to warm up your hamstrings, shoulders, and lower back fully.

Start in Samasthiti. Inhale as you draw your left knee in toward your chest, keeping the knee bent. Roll your left shoulder forward and thread your left elbow under your left knee. Rotate your left shoulder inward, and place your left hand behind your back on top of your sacrum. Drop your right shoulder into internal rotation, and clasp your hands together behind your back. Do not attempt to straighten your left leg if you cannot bind your hands or if your hamstrings are too tight. If your hands are firmly bound, slowly extend your left leg. Drop the head of your left thighbone deeper into its socket, engage your left quadricep, and point your toes. Stabilize your right leg, draw in your lower belly, and gaze forward at a single point. Stay here for five breaths. Return to Samasthiti. Repeat on the right side.

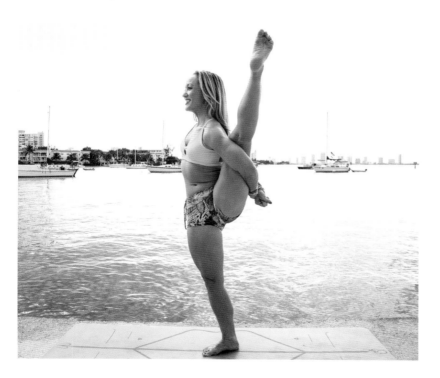

3. *Astavakrasana*—Eight-Angle Pose

This asymmetrical arm balance is a test of balance and nonattachment. While you may be able to hold the balance easily on one side, the other side may prove more challenging. Let go of your attachment and surrender to the journey of putting in the work. You will need all your strength and flexibility to reach full Astavakrasana. Once you have the full expression of the pose, there are endless ways to enter and exit. Let's start off with the easiest entry.

Start in Dandasana. Inhale as you lift your left leg and bend the knee. Aim your left calf muscle around your left shoulder by sending your left knee behind your torso. Bend your left elbow under your left knee, and angle your arm out to the side to maintain good balance. Align your hands on the ground just in front of your hips. Lean forward and lift your hips. Once you find good stability in your arms, lift your right leg and lock your feet around each other. Exhale, stabilize your pelvic floor and prepare to raise up. Inhale as you lift your whole body off the ground. Exhale and bend your elbows to bring your chest down just below your elbows to enter full Astavakrasana. Stay here for five breaths. Inhale as you send your chest forward and drop your hips. Return to Dandasana. Repeat on the right side.

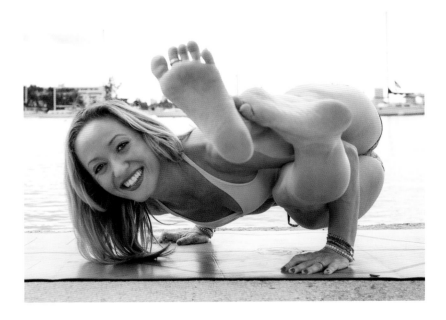

If you don't feel comfortable reaching the full expression of this pose, just go as far you feel do comfortable with and don't force it. Try it a maximum of three times and then move on.

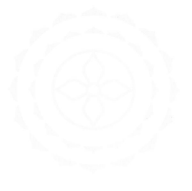

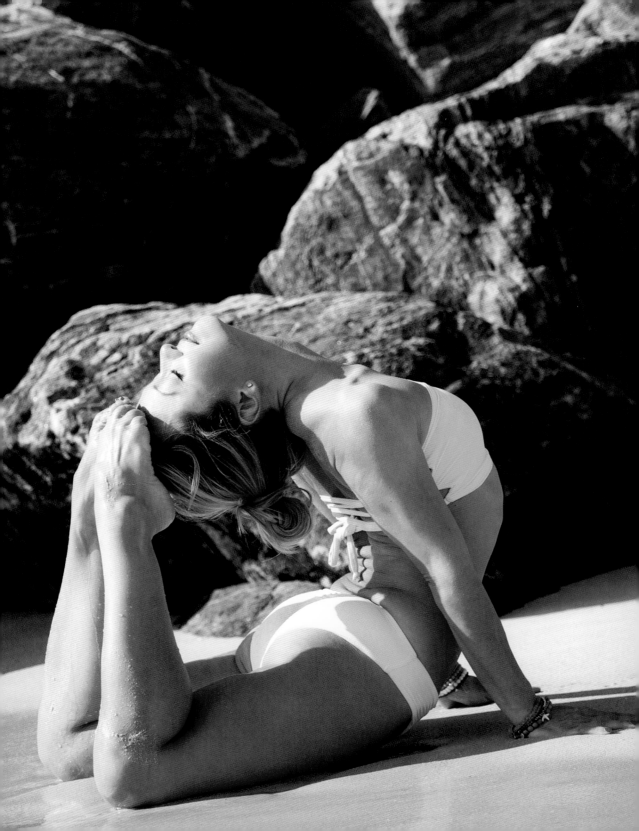

The aspiring yogi may sometimes feel caught in an endless cycle of suffering. From physical pain to emotional frustration to spiritual disillusionment, the spiritual path is not without its potholes and wrong turns. The first step in finding the way out of a trap is to realize that you are trapped. Yoga philosophy brings the obstacles to light, sort of like a GPS app that gives all the possible twists, turns, and detours along a journey. Know the temptations well and you will not be caught by them. Today's yogi assignment is obstacles. Every yoga student will face them, and knowing that is half the battle.

I've faced them all. I've been sick, injured, lazy, and uninspired. I've fallen for false teachers, made errors in judgment, and taken five steps back just after taking five steps forward. I've felt anger, pride, ignorance, depression, and greed, just to name a few. According to Patanjali, there are eleven disturbances (*antarayah*, Yoga Sutra 1.30), five afflictions (*kleshas*, Yoga Sutra 2.3), five vrittis (Yoga Sutra 1.5), and numerous samskaras and other physical accompaniments to the obstacles.

Guruji often talked about the dangers of what he called the six enemies of spiritual practice that surround the heart. They are also sometimes called the six passions and presented as oppositional factors that deter the yogi's mind from a state of nonattachment. The six enemies are known as the *arishadvargas* and are often considered to be some of the main obstacles along the path of yoga. The arishadvargas are lust (*kama*), anger (*krodha*), greed (*lobha*), attachment (*moha*), pride (*mada*), and jealousy (*matsarya*). In addition to these, Patanjali lists a total of fourteen obstacles—nine antarayahs and five kleshas. The nine antarayahs are sickness (*vyadhi*), dullness/stuckness (*styana*), doubt (*samsaya*), negligence (*pramada*), laziness (*alasaya*), sensual pleasure (*avirati*), false preception (*bhranti darshana*), failure to attain firm ground (*alabdhabhumikatva*); and recidivism (*anavasthitatvani*).

The five kleshas are ignorance (*avidya*), ego (*asmita*), attachment to pleasure (*raga*), aversion from pain (*dvesha*), and fear of death (*abhivesha*). The list of obstacles is nearly a perfect description of what it means to be human. Only by facing these destructive tendencies will the yoga student gain access to the spiritual heart. While we could write an entire book on the obstacles, let's take a look at two of the most common enemies to spiritual practice: pride and jealousy.

Sometimes we are too proud to say we're sorry, admit our mistakes, or look like fools. I used to be like that. There was a moment when, after multiple trips to India, I thought I had the inside scoop, that I was special. My pride kicked in, and suddenly I thought I was somebody because I could press up into a handstand. My teachers proceeded to show me otherwise. When I thought I was strong enough, they asked me to be stronger. Where I thought I would be first, they put me last. They sought out and broke down the guard of my ego in every self-satisfied place I had until I realized that I was no better than anyone else and that a handstand isn't a measure of spiritual strength.

Being truly strong has nothing to do with what you can and can't do physically. It has to do with how much you're willing to open your heart. Pride and stubbornness take shape in the Mahabharata as a giant *asura* known as the intoxicator, who has the power to swallow up the entire universe in one gulp. Pride is just like that. It has the power to destroy all your happiness in a flash. The first step down the road of knowledge is to admit that you do not have all the answers and that you need a teacher. There is a fine line between a healthy sense of self-esteem and an inflated ego. Admitting that you're not perfect, that you need help, that you haven't got it all together on your own is sometimes a bigger act of strength and faith than trying to cover up your mess. Having a humble, teachable spirit paves the way for your heart to open and for the power of grace to step in and take the reins of your life. What matters in life is being humble, being kind, and sharing more love. Nobody cares about handstands if you're not a nice person.

Jealousy is a disease of the spirit that emerges from low self-esteem. Persistently focusing on what you lack is a self-directed negativity that stems from a lack of self-worth. I know because I've been there. When I first started practicing, all the yoga postures were so difficult; I struggled with everything. I thought that one day, when I finally got the next pose, I would be whole. It was easy to celebrate people who were far more accomplished than I because they were in another league.

But the practitioners who were around my same level, or just a little further along, drove me nuts. Instead of cultivating a community-oriented attitude, I was consumed with jealousy and competition. Even though I mostly kept this to myself, it still ate away at my heart. I thought their success somehow took mine away. I lost the chance to make lasting friendships. I never believed I was good enough, strong enough, pretty enough. I searched for something to fill the void within.

When you look for your true self in the material world, whether in objects or accomplishments, you always sell yourself short. Choose the higher ground; follow the yogi's path and choose joy (*mudita*) and unlock the keys to true success. Patanjali says that the yogi must cultivate an attitude of joy in the presence of those who are happy and successful (Yoga Sutra 1.33). Joy, like love, never ends—the more you give it to the world, the more there is to go around.

What secrets do you hold under lock and key that silently eat away at your heart and soul? What obstacles of the ego prevent you from opening your heart fully? Be strong enough to break the chains that bind your heart.

HOMEWORK

1. Bring joy to the world. Smile at people, tell them a joke and share laughter, tickle someone, do something silly, laugh at yourself. Share what brings you joy. Or turn negativity around and offer a prayer of joy to someone of whom you are a little jealous. It's humbling to see how hard it is to wish someone joy if we feel jealousy toward them. But offering joyful wishes to others only brings more joy into the world. Give all the joy away, and it will multiply around you.

2. Personalize the obstacles. Make a list of the obstacles you have faced, along with the antidote that would alleviate the spiritual bind. For example, joy is the antidote to jealousy, fulfillment is the antidote to bitterness, faith is the antidote to fear, love is the antidote to hate, and humility is the antidote to ego.

3. Cultivate humility and humor. Being serious is overrated. The ability to laugh at yourself is way more fun—and useful. You'll never be perfect, so let yourself off the hook and have fun, laugh at yourself, and be free.

Humor is a valuable tool on the spiritual path; it comes with humility and is a great antidote to pride. Make funny faces, tell stupid jokes, and laugh. The ability to put your flaws and imperfections on the table and risk being the butt of a joke is a statement of true self-confidence. I never used to be able to laugh at myself, and I used to take everything, including my practice, so seriously. But being serious is just too exhausting to keep up. Laugh and the world laughs with you. Smile and the sun shines on you.

PRACTICE

1. *Ustrasana*—Camel Pose

This backbend is one of the most therapeutic in the yoga practice. It is also accessible to many levels of practitioners and easy to modify. Regular practice of Ustrasana sets up healthy backbending technique and allows you to see deeply into the inner workings of spinal extension. You may discover places of weakness in your muscles and joints. Or you may discover neurological weakness that arises in the form of intense emotions or disturbed breathing. If this happens, it is crucial that you remain calm, check in with your body to protect your joints, and work with a sound technique.

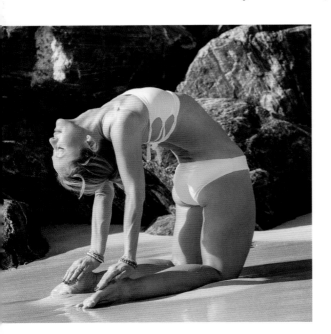

Start off in a kneeling position. Align your knees hip-width apart, and point your toes. Inhale as you place your hands on your hips and draw your subnavel in toward your spine. Engage your back muscles to lift your ribs away from your hips and make space between each of your vertebrae. Send your sternum up toward your chin. Exhale as you send your pelvis forward and bend through each of the joints in your spine to facilitate a gentle spinal extension. Place your hands on the soles of your feet so the heels of your hands align with the heels of your feet and your fingers point toward your toes. Roll your shoulders forward, using internal rotation to elevate the trapezius muscles and support your neck. Root down through the inner edges of your thighs, engage your pelvic floor, and nutate your sacrum to send it forward and slightly up to enter full Ustrasana. Continue lifting your ribs away from your hips. Flexible students should place extra emphasis on the internal strength needed to support the backbend. Gaze toward your nose. Stay here for five breaths.

Inhale and send your hips forward to come up, returning your hands to your waist as you do. Exhale and settle your hips down on your feet again. Rest in Balasana. Repeat Ustrasana one or two times, then jump back to Chaturanga Dandasana. Inhale and come forward to Urdhva Mukha Svanasana; exhale and roll back to Adho Mukha Svanasana.

2. Raja Kapotasana—King Pigeon Pose

Sometimes also called the Royal Pigeon Pose, Raja Kapotasana is a very challenging backbend. If you push too hard to try to force your way in, you will only block yourself. Practicing this pose means making friends with the obstacles that arise along the path to practice.

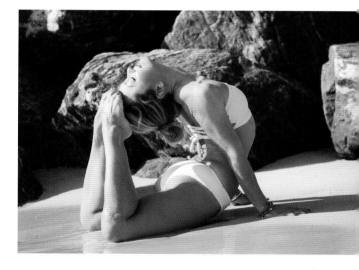

Start off lying on your stomach. Inhale as you slowly start to lift your chest. Place your hands on the ground under your shoulders. Do not try to arch back immediately. Instead, think about creating space between each of the joints of your spine. Lift your shoulders and sternum, maximizing the space between your ribs and hips. Exhale and engage your back muscles to fold into the space between the joints. Bring your shoulders toward your sacrum. Slowly straighten your arms by pushing firmly into the ground. Once your arms are straight, pull slightly with your fingertips and, depending on your level of flexibility, allow your shoulders to move back behind your hands. Soften your glutes, gently allow your legs to bend, and point your toes to enter Raja Kapotasana. Point your toes. Do not try too hard to reach your toes to your head. Instead, keep using the strength of your back to move your head toward your feet. Drop your head back and gaze toward your nose. Stay at your limit for five breaths.

Do not force your feet toward your head. Just accept where you are for today. Exhale and straighten your legs. Keep your arms in position and press up into Urdhva Mukha Svanasana; exhale and roll back to Adho Mukha Svanasana.

3. *Supta Virasana*—Reclining Hero Pose

This pose is a time to turn your attention inward. Used both to prepare for and restore after deep backbends, Supta Virasana focuses on the internal rotation of the hips, a restful state of mind, and a humble heart.

Start off in a kneeling position. Fold your legs under your body and settle your hips onto your feet. Keep your knees and feet together. If your knees feel comfortable, rotate your hips outward, spread your calf muscles out to the side, and widen your feet to just beyond hip-width. Settle your hips between your feet and sink your pelvis down. If your hips do not reach the floor, grab a towel or block to sit on. Place your hands in prayer position at the center of your chest, gently drop your head forward, and gaze toward your nose.

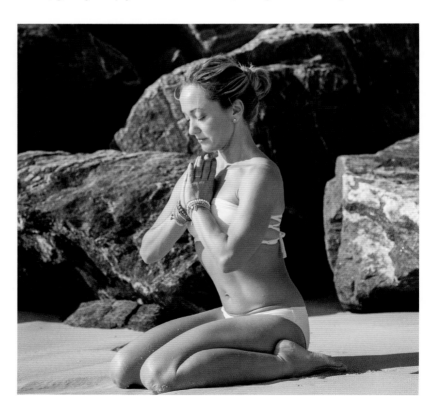

If you have a knee injury that prevents you from closing your knee joints completely, you will need to elevate your hips on a block or bolster to proceed. Exhale as you guide your torso back to a full reclining position, using your hands to help track and support your upper body. Once your shoulders touch the ground, draw your subnavel in toward your spine and place your sacrum on the ground. Draw your knees as close together as possible to facilitate a deeper internal rotation of your hips. Place your hands on your thighs, and gaze toward your nose. Stay here for five to ten breaths.

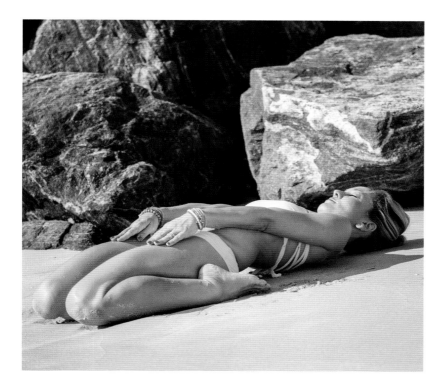

Inhale and come up, using your hands to guide your torso. Inhale and lift up; exhale and jump back to Chaturanga Dandasana. Inhale and come forward to Urdhva Mukha Svanasana; exhale and roll back to Adho Mukha Svanasana.

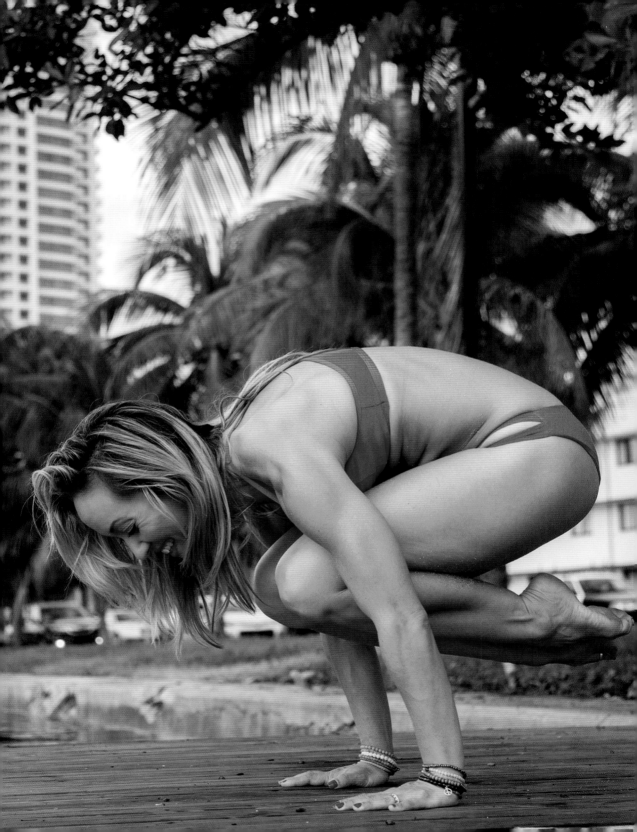

Being Strong
Sthira

The journey of strength has been the most intimate, healing, and challenging lesson for me. I remember the first time I saw the Ashtanga Yoga arm balances; I thought they were magic. Never did I imagine they would be part of my daily practice. I thought of myself as a little girl with wobbly arms and a jiggly butt. Guess what? Not anymore. I'm strong—so much stronger than I ever thought possible. And you know what? So are you! Today's yogi assignment is strength (*sthira*). Strength isn't about pressing up into a handstand (although that is certainly gratifying). It is about finding the rock-solid place of spiritual awareness deep in the center of yourself. Strength is a calm and equanimous mind that remains peaceful and balanced in the face of the inevitable ups and downs of life.

My teachers, Shri K. Pattabhi Jois and R. Sharath Jois, believed in me long before I ever believed in myself. Whenever I felt I had reached a limit and figured that was all I had physically and mentally, they told me to be stronger. Now, after nearly twenty years of practice, I finally am. I remember when I started the practice and everything felt like an uphill struggle—I couldn't do handstands, jump-throughs, or even a headstand. Other people seemed to get strong much faster than I did; I just seemed to sit there and stagnate in heaviness. Lifting up felt as impossible as flying to the moon. None of my success in practice came easily.

The same thing applied to my professional career. When I started teaching, I sent out one hundred emails to studios and got back only a few replies. While I was thankful for the replies I did get, and to the people who supported me from the start, to be met with such a negative response was overwhelming. I wondered if there was some magical formula for success that I just couldn't decipher. When I wanted to publish my first book, numerous agents turned me down, ten told me why I wasn't good enough, and one believed in me and said yes.

All it took was one, and I'm thankful. But facing hundreds of negative replies made me doubt there was space for me in the world. The practice taught me how to be strong and believe in myself against all doubt. I worked tirelessly for my dreams because I believed in them even when no one else did.

For me to find strength, I needed to find faith. When I fell out of a handstand every day for five years, I held on to the faith that my teachers had in me. It was like a promise, and I had to muster great faith to keep practicing. I had no evidence that I would ever succeed; all I had was the choice to believe. I only experienced failure, so the decision to believe in the promise tested the depths of my faith. True strength is spiritual fortitude, and my faith is connected to a deeply personal and profound relationship with God. I finally realized that to be strong I had to find the ultimate source of faith—the Divine.

Faith and strength are equal parts action. Do not rely on luck. Success is for the doggedly determined, the tenacious of spirit, and those strong enough to humbly put in the work. If you don't feel lucky, don't feel like you'll ever win anything, and are never picked out from the crowd, then make your own luck. Don't procrastinate and wait for success to knock on your door. Don't waste your time being bitter about someone else's success, and don't sing about your lack. Have no fear, operate from faith, and take intelligent risks. Be wise, bold, compassionate, and brave. Chip away at that insurmountable mountain one step, one breath at a time. Constantly recalibrate your direction to focus on the value of what you give, not the tally of what you get to take. Be your best self, for yourself, not to please anyone else. Hold yourself to the highest standards, but don't be too perfectionistic. Learn from your mistakes, forgive yourself for failure, and pick yourself back up to try again. Excellence is a sustained attitude of greatness, not an endgame measured by numbers and spreadsheets. Set your aim with perseverance, grit, and unwavering faith. Believe in yourself and never give up.

1. Decide not to quit. At least half of being strong is making a decision to never quit. Is there a dream you have quietly abandoned that you could recommit yourself to today? Ask yourself what action you can take today to make one small step toward accomplishing your dreams.

2. Do strength drills. If you want to be physically strong, you will have to work for it. Commit to repeating the poses outlined in this chapter every day for one year. It will only take you five minutes and will add a new level of physical strength to your practice.

3. Improve emotional strength. Set emotional boundaries clearly, lovingly, and patiently. Give up all vindictiveness, uproot all bitterness, burn all anger. But be resolute about who you are. Don't settle for anything that sets you up as a second-rate citizen worth less than your true value. Choose one toxic situation you are finally strong enough to walk away from, or choose to speak up for yourself when someone crosses a line. Make this concrete by writing about it in your journal, and note today's date as the turning point when you decided to build your life on the rock of self-confidence that comes from knowing exactly who you are. You are strong. You are whole and complete. You are a bright and beautiful spirit. You have been born to share a unique and valuable contribution with the world. Never forget it!

1. *Utthita Chaturanga Dandasana*—Plank Pose

PRACTICE

Utthita Chaturanga Dandasana is an integral part of building strength. I love all types of plank poses and do them every day as part of my strength routine. Utthita Chaturanga Dandasana is accessible for nearly everyone and can be used to both strengthen and rehabilitate the shoulders.

Start off on your hands and knees. Place your hands shoulder-width apart and your knees together. Align your shoulders over your palms, and keep your fingers in a neutral position. Draw in your navel and subnavel, and tuck your lower ribs in toward the center line. Widen your shoulder blades and lengthen your tailbone. Inhale as you engage your lower abdominal muscles, and tighten your whole torso by activating your core muscles to lift into Utthita Chaturanga Dandasana. Press into the ground with the strength of your shoulders to widen your shoulder blades as much as possible. Keep your weight in the balls of your feet, draw your thighs together, and gently activate your glutes. Gaze between your hands. Stay here for five breaths. Sink your knees back to the ground, and rest in Balasana. Repeat three times.

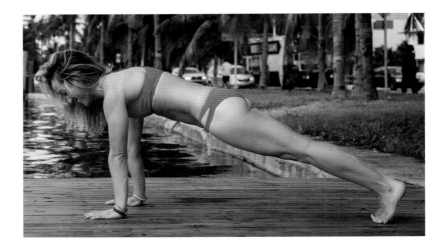

2. *Brahmacharyasana*—L-sit

The L-sit is an integral part of every seated jump-through and is essential for building strength. You may feel like you will never lift up all the way, but the L-sit can be modified to make it accessible for everyone.

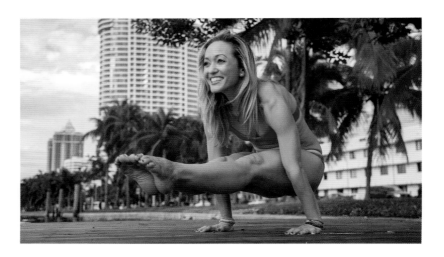

Start in Dandasana. Inhale and make space behind your pubic bone as you fold slightly forward. Place your hands on the ground at midthigh (in front of your hips and behind your knees). Exhale and send your shoulders over your palms. Point the crown of your head toward your toes. Engage your lower abdominal muscles and draw in your lower ribs. Activate your quadriceps, and flex your feet. Inhale and straighten your arms to lift your hips off the ground. Drag your hips back as you send your shoulders forward. Keep your ribs and hips as close together as possible. Eventually, your feet will lift up as you send your hips back, coming into the full L-sit. Gaze at the tip of your nose. Avoid kicking or jumping your feet up, and just lift your hips, even if your feet do not come off the ground. Stay here for five breaths. Lower your hips and return to Dandasana. Repeat three times.

3. *Lolasana*—Pendant Pose

This humble lift is harder than a handstand. If you have the strength to keep both feet off the ground for five solid breaths, then you have the strength to master most arm balances in any yoga practice. But if you lack the strength, you may feel—as I did when I started—that your butt will just never get off the ground. With patient, persistent practice, you *will* get stronger.

Start off on your hands and knees. Place your hands shoulder-width apart. Align your shoulders over your palms, and keep your fingers in a neutral position. Draw in your navel and subnavel, and tuck your lower ribs in toward the center line. Widen your shoulder blades and lengthen your tailbone. Draw your knees forward, keeping your feet and knees together. Point your toes and bring your knees between your arms. Be sure your knees are in front of your wrists. Inhale as you engage your pelvic floor, activate your lower abdominal muscles, firm your shoulder girdle, and lift both feet to come into Lolasana. Gaze at the floor just in front of your fingers. Stay here for five breaths. Lower your hips and come down to rest. Repeat three times. If you cannot lift both feet, hold the preparatory position and lift one foot at a time, but do not jump or kick up.

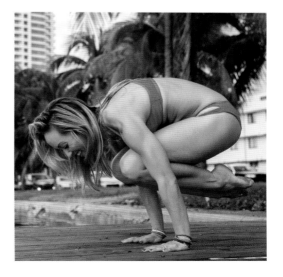

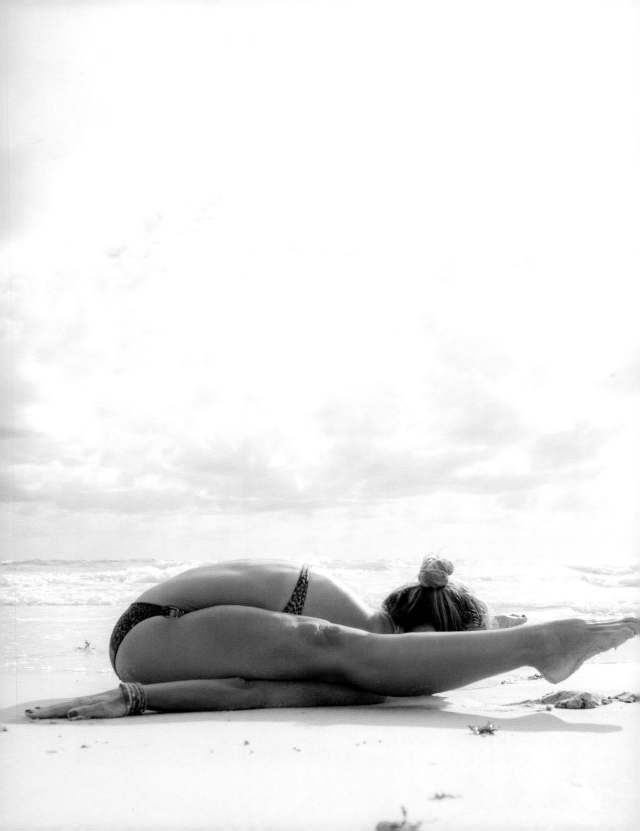

Day 30 Seeking Refuge in Divine Shelter
Sharanam

n our own way and in our own time, we are all searching for home. We all need a feeling of belonging and a sense of lasting peace. We are beings of light and love, yet we are all scarred, wounded, hurting, suffering, and fighting our own epic emotional battles. Our only shelter is in the wings of grace. There is no permanent happiness in the material world. There is no firm ground to stand on amid the shifting sands of time. Everything is temporary; every moment is fleeting.

Today's yogi assignment is refuge (*sharanam*). The only real place to seek refuge is in the center of your heart through complete surrender. *Sha* stands for the humility to ask for help and the grace that sets you free from all human obstacles. *Ra* stands for the liberating direct experience of God, contains the acoustic root of fire, and symbolizes Divine light and fire. *Nam* stands for the deep peace and inner silence that is the domain of God. Akin to the noumenal, *nam* also stands for God's word and the name of God, through which we can directly experience the revelation of ultimate truth. Another way of understanding the concept of sharanam is to think of it as the moment when you are overwhelmed with the unparalleled power, magnitude, and beauty of God's presence and have no choice but to surrender.

Patanjali's Yoga Sutras present the notion of sharanam as Ishvara Pranidhana over a series of seven sutras (Yoga Sutras 1.23–29). Translated as "devotion to the Lord," Ishvara Pranidhana is the active state of seeking refuge. More than a religious dogma or legalistic structure, it happens through the direct experience of God's greatness. Only then will yoga practitioners truly devote themselves to worship with humility and reverence. Devotion happens when you love something or someone. You love what you are devoted to. But you cannot love something truly until you have experienced it. Yoga gives you a forum to directly experience God within yourself and thereby cultivate an attitude of surrender.

Shri K. Pattabhi Jois always said, "Do your practice, think about God." It is only after nearly twenty years of practice that I fully begin to understand the power and depth of his simple statement.

I was not raised with any religion, nor did I believe in the principle of God for a long time. In fact, the mere mention of God used to make me antsy, and I abhorred the use of the masculine article *He* to refer to God. But now I can say that I have experienced God directly and that, through His greatness, I have known more freedom than I ever thought possible. For me, it is no longer a question of whether or not there is a God, because I know Him, have a relationship with Him, and love Him. Yoga is a revolutionary tool that gives every single person the chance to know God directly. You don't need to pass any tests, memorize any ancient books, or go through any religious rituals. All you need to do is breathe and turn your mind inward, and the truth will reveal itself to you.

According to traditional yoga philosophy, only the holy sound OM comes remotely close to communicating the greatness of God. OM is the sacred symbol for God, the truest name of God that we have. Think back to your first yoga class and remember the vibration of OM that touched your heart beyond thoughts and concepts. It is the vibration of stillness that rings out from silence, the sound that echoes to the depths of the universe. The purity of its vibration can bring you to an experience of Divine greatness. Your mind stills. Your heart opens. Your spirit sings. And the resonance opens a channel to the direct experience of God.

The sacred symbol OM (ॐ) can be traced back to the ancient Rig Veda, from the second millennium B.C.E. It is a mystic syllable for the name of God, the vibration that lies underneath and connects the entire universe. The Upanishads say that the essence of all things is contained within OM. The mystic symbol is composed of three syllables, which explains why you often see it written as AUM. In Sanskrit, the vowel *o* is a diphthong compound of *a + u*, making the sound much like one long O and not two separate A and U sounds. The A symbolizes the waking state (*jagrat*), the most common human experience. In this state, consciousness is turned outward through the gates of the senses. The U symbolizes the dream state (*svapna*) in which the consciousness is turned inward to a personal reality. The M symbolizes the dreamless sleep state (*sushupti*). Everyone experiences these three states. The dot symbolizes the resonance, the *turiya* state, a fourth state of consciousness only available to yogis and spiritual seekers. The mind is in a calm, equanimous state, free from obstacles and fully liberated.

Every person has a spiritual yearning in his or her heart. It registers differently for everyone, but we all feel it. Some people experience this quiet yearning as a quest for adventure, a desire to be loved, a relentless drive for achievement, or an overwhelming sadness. This spiritual anguish is part of what it means to be human. I felt it as depression, a sense of separation, and a residual angst that could not find rest. True home is not a physical place or even a group of people. Your true home is in the spirit. Find the path to the world within and discover the highest truth. There is a brightness in you that yearns to shine. The heart is the key to unlocking the star within you. If you are acting with love, then everything is in your favor. If you are acting without love, then even if you are the most powerful person, you are weak. There is a quiet voice of wisdom that speaks to you from your heart center. Listen from your heart and that voice will call you to your spiritual home. It says, *I am here. I have always been with you. There is no place where I am not. There is no time when I am not.* With faith, follow the subtle glow that is the seed of your new dawn. Seek your home in the world within, and it will be revealed.

1. Find the resonance of OM. Take a comfortable seated position in a quiet place. Close your eyes. Begin with a calm and equanimous mind. Place your hands in prayer position at the center of your chest. Inhale fully. Exhale the sound OM. Let it resonate all the way to the end of your exhalation. Repeat this three times. Remain seated and observe the inner body.

2. Hear God's voice. Take a comfortable seated position in a quiet place. Close your eyes. Begin with a calm and equanimous mind. Sit in silence for a minimum of five breaths. Place your mind's point of attention at your spiritual heart center, in the space behind your sternum. Listen for a quiet voice of wisdom that speaks to you through stillness.

3. Surrender. Take a comfortable seated position in a quiet place. Close your eyes. Begin with a calm and equanimous mind. Sit in silence for a minimum of five breaths. Place your hands in prayer position at the center of your chest. Surrender your will to God's will and give Him permission to take the driver's seat in your life for today.

HOMEWORK

PRACTICE

1. Ekam

The first breath of the practice always starts with the first position of Surya Namaskar A (Sun Salutation), known in Ashtanga simply as Ekam. The simple act of raising the arms above the head embodies the subtle simplicity of the yoga journey. Ekam, the first breath, is the initiation into the spiritual heart of the practice. Like the first word of a story, the first breath of the practice is like the breath of life. The number one is also symbolic of the singularity of God.

Start in Samasthiti. Inhale as you raise your hands above your head and press the palms together. Align your body along the center line. Draw in your lower ribs slightly, engage your core muscles, and suck in your navel to support your spine. Rotate your shoulders outward, and straighten your arms completely. Firm your quadriceps, and maximize the space between your ribs and hips. Gaze up at your thumbs. After one deep inhalation, you are ready to proceed to Surya Namaskar A (see The Power of Ashtanga Yoga I for a complete discussion of the Sun Salutations).

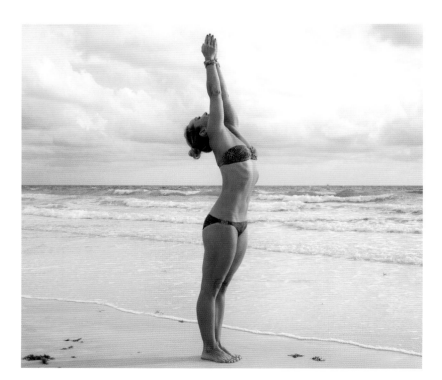

2. *Kurmasana*—Tortoise Pose

This pose requires faith, surrender, and devotion. It is common in the Ashtanga Yoga method to have your teacher physically adjust you in Kurmasana. During these adjustments, your emotional and physical limitations are often met. Only with faith and surrender to your teacher will Kurmasana start to feel comfortable.

Jump forward from Adho Mukha Svanasana with your legs. Walk your feet as far in front of your hands as possible. Stack your thighs on top of your shoulders. Reach your hands and arms under the thighs, slightly back and to the side in a diagonal from your shoulders. Point your fingers away from the shoulders, straighten your arms, and place your palms down to the sides of your hips. Settle your pelvis to the ground. Straighten your legs as you reach your chest forward. Keep your thighs as close to your shoulders as possible and avoid widening your legs. Engage your chest and shoulders to protect your sternum. Slide your elbows back and through your thighs. With each breath, sink lower until your forehead, chin, or shoulders touch the ground. Fully straighten your legs and eventually lift your heels off the ground. Stay for five breaths. Slowly lift yourself up and jump back to Chaturanga Dandasana. Inhale and come forward to Urdhva Mukha Svanasana; exhale and roll back to Adho Mukha Svanasana. If you do not feel ready to try this pose, substitute Bhujapidasana.

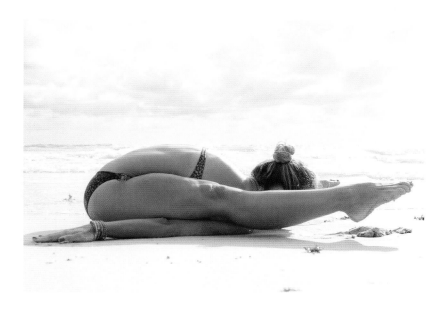

3. *Eka Pada Raja Kapotasana*—One-Legged King Pigeon Pose

This pose will bring up your need to surrender. It is a deep, asymmetrical backbend that can take you off center if you don't have a stable sense of your core. There are two ways to enter Eka Pada Raja Kapotasana; for today, let's look at the one that requires more faith.

Start in Adho Mukha Svanasana. Inhale as you step your right foot forward. Bend your right knee to close the joint, and fold your right foot in by your pubic bone. Point your toes. Settle your hips on the ground and square them forward. Straighten your left leg and point your toes. Inhale as you take your hands to your waist. Lift your ribs away from your hips, and maximize the space between your vertebrae. Exhale and engage your back muscles to fold into a spinal extension. Take your hands to prayer position. Bend your left knee gently. Inhale and lift your hands over your head, reaching toward your left foot. Hold your left foot with both hands and drop your head back to enter full Eka Pada Raja Kapotasana. If you cannot reach your foot, simply leave your hands in the air and reach in the direction of your foot. Stay here for five breaths.

Slowly place your hands on the ground and step back to Chaturanga Dandasana. Inhale and come forward to Urdhva Mukha Svanasana; exhale and roll back to Adho Mukha Svanasana. Repeat on the right side.

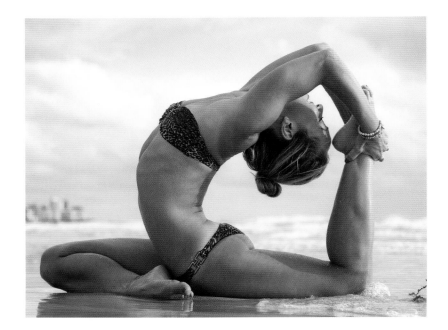

4. *Yoga Mudra*—Sacred Seal

Yoga Mudra is usually placed at the end of your practice to symbolize sealing in the deep spiritual work of each practice session.

Start in Dandasana. Fold your legs into either Comfortable Seated Pose or Padmasana. Reach behind your back to grasp the opposite elbows. If you are comfortably in Padmasana, reach your left hand to your left foot and your right hand to your right foot for Baddha Padmasana. From whichever version of the pose is accessible to you today, fold forward to enter Yoga Mudra. Reach either your forehead or your chin to the ground. Stay here for ten breaths. Inhale and come up to Padmasana.

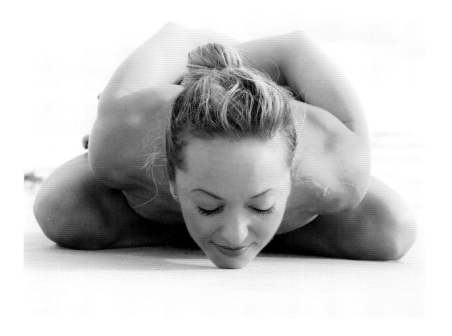

Pose Glossary

This glossary presents all the poses included in the book, as well as some other common or transitional poses that are mentioned in the text.

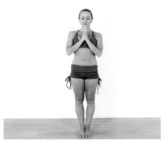

1. *Samasthiti*—Equal Standing Pose

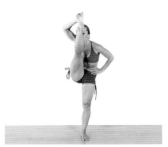

2. *Trikonasana A*—Triangle Pose

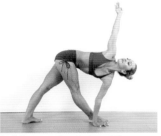

3. *Trikonasana B* or *Parivrtta Trikonasana*—Revolved or Twisted Triangle Pose

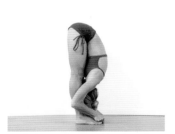

4. *Padangusthasana*—Hand-to-Big-Toe Pose

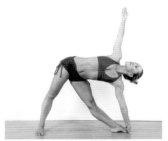

5a. *Utthita Hasta Padangusthasana A*—Extended Hand-to-Big-Toe Pose A

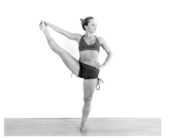

5b. *Utthita Hasta Padangusthasana B*—Extended Hand-to-Big-Toe Pose B

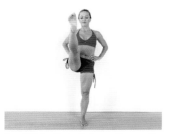

5c. *Utthita Hasta Padangusthasana C*—Extended Hand-to-Big-Toe Pose C

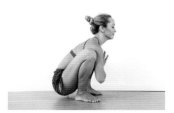

6. *Malasana*—Garland or Mala Pose

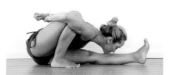

7a. *Marichyasana A*—Pose Dedicated to the Sage Marichi A

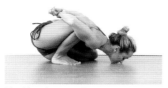

7b. *Marichyasana B*—Pose Dedicated to the Sage Marichi B

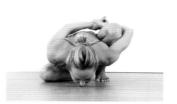

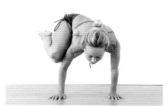

7c. *Marichyasana C*—Pose Dedicated to the Sage Marichi C

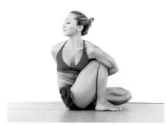

7d. *Marichyasana D*—Pose Dedicated to the Sage Marichi D

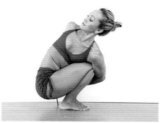

8. *Pasasana*—Noose Pose

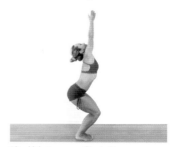

9. *Parsva Bakasana*—Side Crane Pose

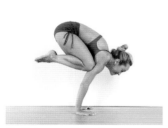

10. *Bakasana*—Crane Pose

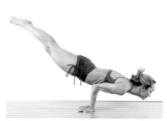

11. *Mayurasana*—Peacock Pose

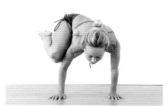

12. *Utkatasana*—Chair Pose

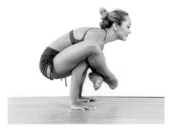

13a. *Bhujapidasana A*—Shoulder Pressing Pose A

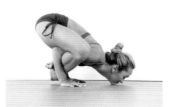

13b. *Bhujapidasana B*—Shoulder Pressing Pose B

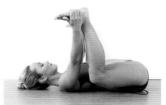

14. *Ananda Balasana*—Happy Baby Pose

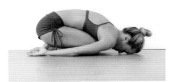

15. *Balasana*—Child's Pose

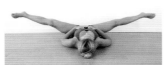

16. *Supta Samakonasana*—
Reclining Straddle or Reclining
Straight Angle Pose

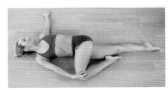

17. *Supta Matsyendrasana*—
Supine Spinal Twist or Reclining Twist

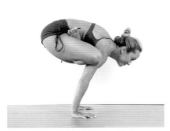

18. *Urdhva Kukkutasana*—Flying
Rooster or Upward-Facing Cock Pose

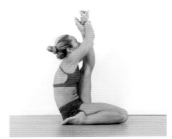

19. *Krounchasana*—Heron Pose

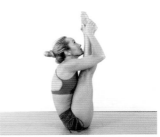

20. *Urdhva Mukha Paschimattanasana*—
Upward-Facing Intense Stretch or
Upward-Facing Forward Bend Pose

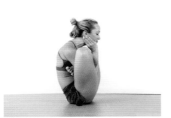

21. *Garbha Pindasana*—
Womb Embryo Pose

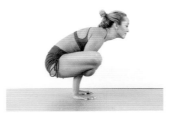

22. *Kukkutasana*—
Rooster or Cock Pose

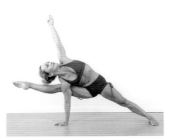

23. *Visvamitrasana*—Visvamitra's Pose

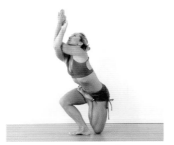

24. *Vatayanasana*—Horse Pose

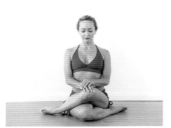

25. *Sukha Gomukhasana*—
Relaxed Cow-Face Pose

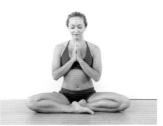

26. *Sukhasana*—
Comfortable Seated Pose

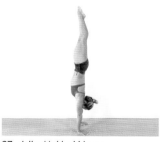

27. *Adho Mukha Vrksasana*—
Straight Line Handstand

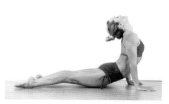

28. *Urdhva Mukha Svanasana*—
Upward-Facing Dog Pose

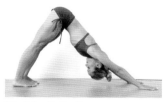

29. *Adho Mukha Svanasana*—
Downward-Facing Dog Pose

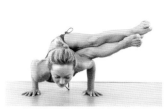

30. *Koundinyasana*—Pose Dedicated
to the Sage Koundinya

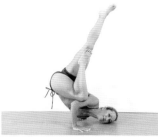

31. *Devaduuta Panna Asana*—
Fallen Angel Pose

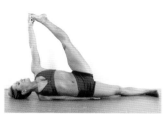

32. *Samanasana*—Balancing Prana
or Side Lying Pose

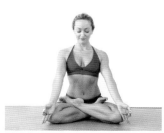

33. *Padmasana*—Lotus Pose

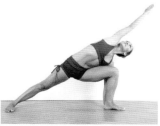

34. *Utthita Parsvakonasana A*—
Extended Side-Angle Pose

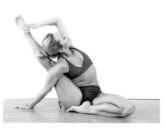

35. *Parivrtta Surya Yantrasana*—
Compass Pose

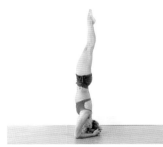

36. *Baddha Hasta Sirsasana A*—
Bound Hand Headstand A

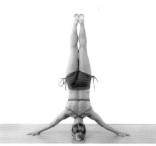

37. *Mukta Hasta Sirsasana C*—
Unsupported Headstand C

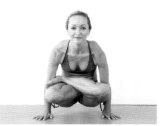

38. *Utpluthih* or *Tolasana*—
Sprung Up or Scales Pose

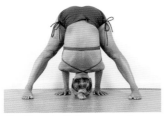

**39a. *Prasarita Padottanasana A—*
Wide-Legged Forward Bend A**

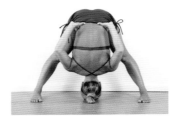

**39b. *Prasarita Padottanasana B—*
Wide-Legged Forward Bend B**

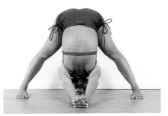

**39c. *Prasarita Padottanasana C—*
Wide-Legged Forward Bend C**

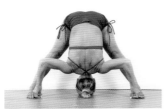

**39d. *Prasarita Padottanasana D—*
Wide-Legged Forward Bend D**

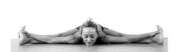

**40a. *Upavistha Konasana A—*
Wide Angle Seated Forward Bend A**

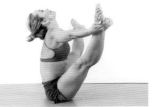

**40b. *Upavistha Konasana B—*
Wide Angle Seated Forward Bend B**

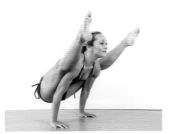

41. *Tittibhasana A—*Firefly Pose A

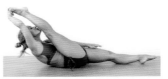

**42a. *Supta Padangusthasana A—*
Reclining Hand-to-Big-Toe Pose A**

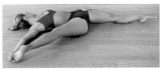

**42b. *Supta Padangusthasana B—*
Reclining Hand-to-Big-Toe Pose B**

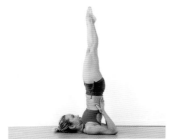

**43. *Salami Sarvangasana—*
Shoulderstand or All-Limbs Pose**

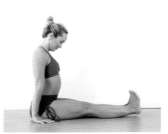

44. *Dandasana—*Staff Pose

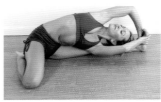

45. *Parighasana—*Gate Pose

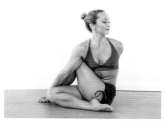

46. *Ardha Matsyendrasana*—
Half Lord of the Fishes Pose

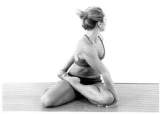

47. *Bharadvajasana*—Pose Dedicated
to the Sage Bharadvaja

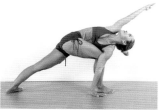

48. *Parivrtta Parsvakonasana* or *Utthita Parsvakonasana B*—Revolved Extended Side-Angle Pose or Extended Side-Angle Pose

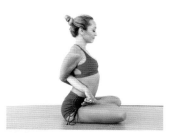

49. *Baddha Padmasana*—
Bound Lotus Pose

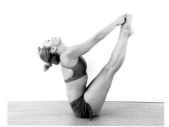

50. *Ubhaya Padangusthasana*—
Double Big Toe Pose

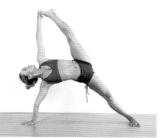

51. *Vashisthasana*—Side Plank Pose

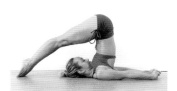

52. *Halasana*—Plow Pose

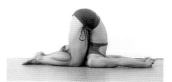

53. *Karnapidasana*—Ear Pressure Pose

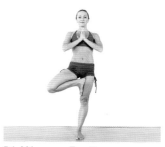

54. *Vrksasana*—Tree Pose

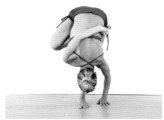

55. *Ardha Baddha Padmottanasana*—
Half Bound Lotus Standing Forward Fold

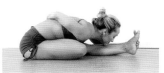

56. *Ardha Baddha Paschimattanasana*—
Half Bound Lotus Forward Fold

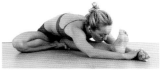

57. *Janu Sirsasana A*—
Head-to-Knee Pose

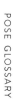

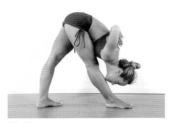

58. *Parsvottanasana*—
Intense Side Stretch Pose

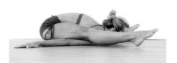

59. *Kurmasana*—Tortoise Pose

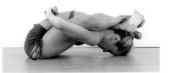

60. *Supta Kurmasana*—
Sleeping Tortoise Pose

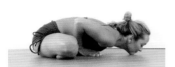

61a. *Baddha Konasana A*—
Bound Angle Pose or Cobbler Pose A

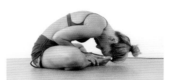

61b. *Baddha Konasana B*—
Bound Angle Pose or Cobbler Pose B

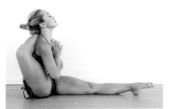

62a. *Eka Pada Sirsasana A*—
Foot-behind-the-Head Pose A

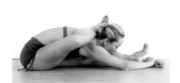

62b. *Eka Pada Sirsasana B*—
Foot-behind-the-Head Pose B

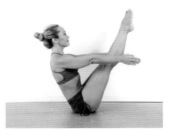

63. *Navasana*—Boat Pose

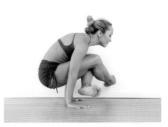

64. *Astau*—"Eight" or Lift Up

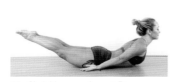

65. *Shalabhasana*—Locust Pose

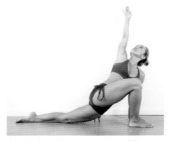

66. *Utthan Pristhasana*—Lizard Pose

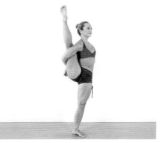

67. *Svarga Dvijasana*—
Bird of Paradise Pose

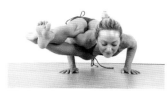

68. *Astavakrasana*—Eight-Angle Pose

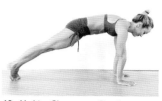

69. *Utthita Chaturanga Dandasana*—Plank Pose or Extended Four-Pointed Staff Pose

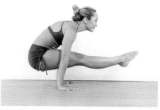

70. *Bramacharyasana*—L-sit or Celibate's Pose

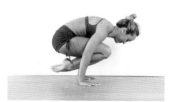

71. *Lolasana*—Pendant Pose

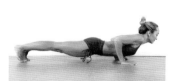

72. *Chaturanga Dandasana*—Four-Pointed Staff Pose

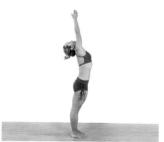

73. *Ekam*—The First Breath

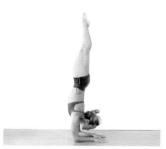

74. *Pinchamayurasana*—Feathered Peacock Pose

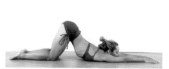

75. *Uttana Shishosana*—Extended Puppy Pose

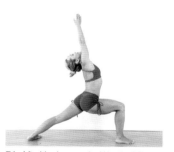

76. *Virabhadrasana A*—Warrior I Pose

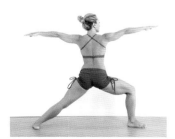

77. *Virabhadrasana B*—Warrior II Pose

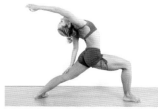

78. *Viparita Virabhadrasana*—Reverse Warrior Pose

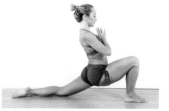

79a. *Anjaneyasana A*—Low Lunge or Pose Dedicated to Anjaneya, a name of Hanuman, A

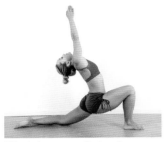

79b. *Anjaneyasana B*—Low Lunge or Pose Dedicated to Anjaneya, a name of Hanuman, B

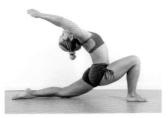

79c. *Anjaneyasana C*—Low Lunge or Pose Dedicated to Anjaneya, a name of Hanuman, C

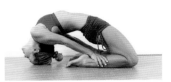

80. *Laghuvajrasana*—Little Thunderbolt Pose

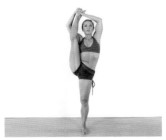

81a. *Hanumanasana A*—Pose Dedicated to Hanuman A, or the Splits

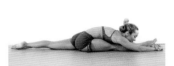

81b. *Hanumanasana B*—Pose Dedicated to Hanuman B, or the Splits

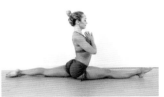

81c. *Hanumanasana C*—Pose Dedicated to Hanuman C, or the Splits

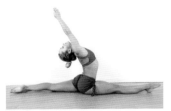

82a. *Trivikramasana A*—Standing Splits or Pose Dedicated to Trivikrama A

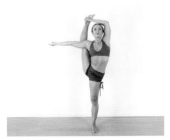

82b. *Trivikramasana B*—Standing Splits or Pose Dedicated to Trivikrama B

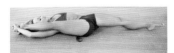

83. *Supta Trivikramasana*—Reclining Splits or Reclining Pose Dedicated to Trivikrama

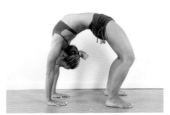

84. *Urdhva Dhanurasana*—Upward Bow Pose or Lifted Wheel Pose

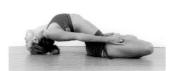

85. *Matsyasana*—Fish Pose

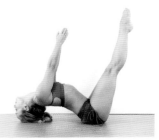

86. *Uttana Padasana*—Raised Leg Pose

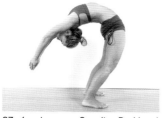

87. *Anuvittasana*—Standing Backbend

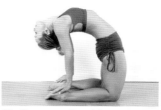

88. *Ustrasana*—Camel Pose

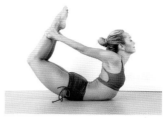

89. *Dhanurasana*—Wheel Pose

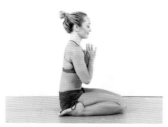

90. *Virasana*—Hero's Pose

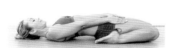

91. *Supta Virasana*— Reclining Hero's Pose

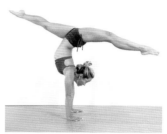

92. *Urdhva Hasta Hanumanasana*— Handstand Splits

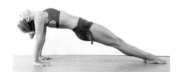

93. *Purvottanasana*— Upward Plank Pose

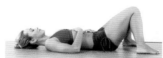

94. Constructive Rest Pose

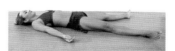

95. *Savasana*—Corpse Pose or "Take Rest"

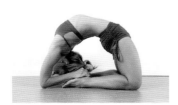

96a. *Kapotasana A*—Pigeon Pose A

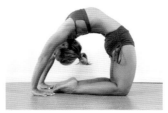

96b. *Kapotasana B*—Pigeon Pose B

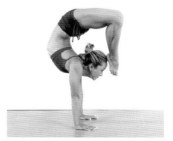

97. *Vrschikasana*— Scorpion Handstand Pose

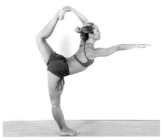

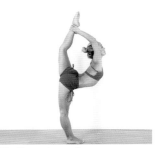

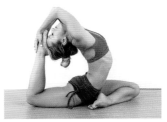

98a. *Natarajasana A—*
Lord of the Dance Pose A

98b. *Natarajasana B—*
Lord of the Dance Pose B

99. *Eka Pada Raja Kapotasana—*
One-Legged King Pigeon Pose

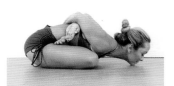

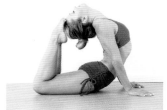

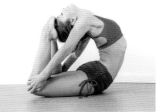

100. *Yoga Mudra—*
Sacred Seal or Yoga Seal

101a. *Raja Kapotasana A—*
King or Royal Pigeon Pose A

101b. *Raja Kapotasana B—*
King or Royal Pigeon Pose B

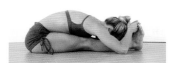

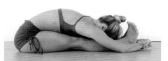

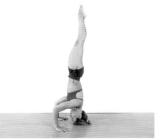

102a. *Paschimattanasana A—*
Intense West Facing Pose or
Intense Forward Fold A

102d. *Paschimattanasana D—*
Intense West Facing Pose or
Intense Forward Fold D

103. *Mukta Hasta Sirsasana A—*
Tripod or Unsupported Headstand A

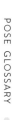

About the Author

Kino MacGregor is a lifelong yoga practitioner who believes that every person can unlock their highest potential through the practice of yoga. As a person of deep faith and personal dedication, she is a messenger of hope and healing to students worldwide. She is known for her sense of humor, love of beauty, and boundless energy. She likes to think of herself as a handstand lover, a beach bum, and just an ordinary girl who found peace through the miracle of grace. But more than anything, Kino is a student of yoga who starts each day in the sacred space of sadhana, in communion with the true light within. All that she shares flows out of the innermost sanctuary of the Divine within her heart.

Kino is an international yoga teacher, author of four books, producer of six Ashtanga Yoga DVDs, writer, vlogger, world traveler, co-founder of OmStars Yoga TV Network, co-founder of Miami Life Center, and co-creator of the Yoga Pro Wheel. She is one of the few people in the world of yoga to embrace both the traditional teaching of India's historic past and the popular contemporary social-media channels. You can find her teaching classes and workshops all over the world, on Kino Yoga Instagram with over one million followers, on her OmStars channel, and on Kino Yoga YouTube channel with more than 100 million views. With nearly twenty years of experience in Ashtanga Yoga, she is one of a select group of people to receive the certification to teach Ashtanga Yoga by its founder Shri K. Pattabhi Jois in Mysore, India, and to practice into the Fifth Series of Ashtanga Yoga.

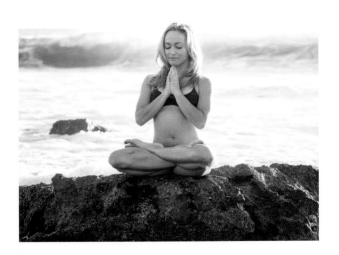